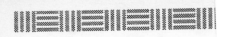

THE ALMOST
MEATLESS
DIET BOOK

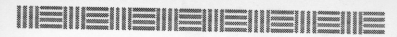

also by Martha Rose Shulman

THE VEGETARIAN FEAST

GARLIC COOKERY

HERBS AND HONEY COOKERY

SPICY VEGETARIAN FEASTS

FAST VEGETARIAN FEASTS

GOURMET VEGETARIAN FEASTS

CHEZ MARTHA ROSE

MEDITERRANEAN LIGHT

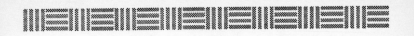

THE ALMOST MEATLESS DIET BOOK

MARTHA ROSE SHULMAN

Delicious Diet Plans
for
Long-lasting Weight Loss

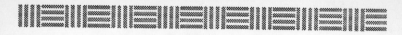

First published 1990 by
MACMILLAN LONDON LIMITED
4 Little Essex Street London WC2R 3LF
and Basingstoke

Associated companies in Auckland, Delhi, Dublin, Gaborone, Hamburg,
Harare, Hong Kong, Johannesburg, Kuala Lumpur, Lagos, Manzini,
Melbourne, Mexico City, Nairobi, New York, Singapore and Tokyo.

ISBN 0-333-52500-0

A CIP catalogue record for this book is available from the
British Library.

Typeset by Matrix, 21 Russell Street, London WC2

Printed in Great Britain by Billings Book Plan

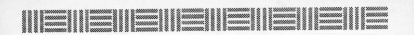

To Abner Stein

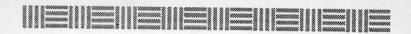

Acknowledgements

I would like to thank Kyle Cathie for helping to bring about this book, and Brenda Thomson for her fine editing skills.

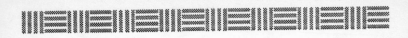

Contents

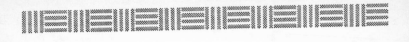

Introduction

A sensible diet

Experience has taught me that the only way to lose weight and keep it off is to lose it gradually by eating a balanced, satisfying, low-fat diet and to combine this healthy eating with regular exercise. Crash diets are diets of deprivation and, precisely for this reason, they usually don't work. Our bodies are as primitive now as they were in the Stone Age, when men and women subsisted on very little. During times of famine the body adapted by slowing down its metabolism. It does the same thing now if it is undernourished, no matter what the reason. And when it does that, weight loss is difficult. Also, as anyone who has ever been on a crash diet knows, once you go off you overcompensate and usually gain back more weight than you lost.

This, then, is not a crash diet. Inspired by the wide variety of produce, fish and fowl that my local Paris markets offer, it is based on my own diet, which is a low-fat, primarily vegetarian one. More and more people tell me they are eating little or no red meat or pork, so these low-fat, nearly meatless diet plans should appeal to many of you. No steak or chips here, but a lot of fresh salads and light soups, simply cooked chicken, rabbit and fish with light sauces, whole grains, beans and tofu.

The diet is naturally low in fats, which contain the most difficult-to-burn calories. Oils, lard, vegetable fat, margarine and butter are pure fat; but some of these are less calorific or less harmful than others because of their chemical structure. Liquid vegetable oils are less saturated than solid fats and easier to metabolise. They're less calorific and not so hard on your arteries. Red meat and pork is loaded with hidden saturated fat, even when you cut away the trim, and by eliminating it and keeping your consumption of high-fat dairy products to a minimum, you can cut your calorie intake drastically. Adapting these eating habits is one of the easiest ways I can think of to lose weight and maintain a lean figure.

Grains, wholemeal breads, pulses, vegetables, fruits, low-fat dairy products, many kinds of fish, rabbit, and chicken and turkey without the skin are very low in fats. So mine is a diet that emphasises these items.

All of the fresh produce, grains, beans and wholemeal breads make this

1

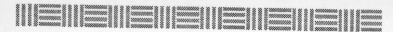

diet a very high-fibre one. The dishes fill you up quickly without weighing you down. And because these foods have so much good texture, you tend to chew them more, which causes you to eat more slowly. The more slowly you eat, the less you will eat.

Vegetables take on a new dimension once you begin to look at them as a real food and not just a side dish. There is so much good flavour here that, even if you're used to eating red meat regularly, you'll feel satisfied. Indeed, when I serve a meal without meat, most of my dinner guests never realise that it's vegetarian.

The starch myth

Most of the calories in grains, wholemeal breads, pulses and vegetables come from *complex carbohydrates*, more commonly known as starches. Unfortunately, foods like grains, breads, pasta and potatoes, which contain high amounts of complex carbohydrates, are popularly regarded as 'fattening'. This couldn't be further from the truth. Gram for gram, complex carbohydrates have the same number of calories as protein. And complex carbohydrates are a much more efficient form of energy for the body than proteins. They are the easiest calories for the body to burn, and the first ones to go. Unfortunately, they have become a diminishing element in our diet over the years, as high-fat meats and nutritionally worthless junk foods and soft drinks have taken over. But with this diet they become the focus, as they should be, and the main source of energy and calories. Foods high in complex carbohydrates are filling, satisfying and nutritious. They are fattening only if you top them with fats such as butter or cheese.

Keeping fats down and protein up

Of course, it's easy to eat a *bad* vegetarian diet, if you eat nothing but crisps, raisins and nuts, or if you have too much of one kind of food. Many people embark upon vegetarianism without knowing the fundamental principles of nutrition and end up compromising their health. Or they end up gaining weight, because they eat too many highly saturated nuts, or concentrate on high-fat dairy products. Dairy products contain excellent protein, but also a great deal of fat: 75 per cent of the calories in Cheddar cheese, for example, are fat calories.

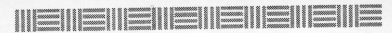

Obtaining enough protein from a vegetarian diet is in fact easy once you understand the principles of food combining. A protein is a long chain of molecules called amino acids. Eight of those amino acids, called *essential amino acids*, must be obtained from food. The eight amino acids exist in fairly equal proportion in meat, fish, dairy products, eggs, tofu and soy beans. Grains and pulses, however, are high in some amino acids and low in others. Taken together, though, or with dairy products, these foods provide what is called *complete protein* – i.e. they provide us with all eight of the essential amino acids. Only complete protein is usable by the body.

This kind of food combining is called *protein complementarity*. All the menus in this book are designed with protein complementarity in mind. Sometimes the complete protein might not come until the end of the meal, in the form of a dessert containing dairy products, but it will always be there.

Here are some simple guidelines for obtaining enough protein from a vegetarian diet. Choosing from any one of them will provide you with complete protein:

- Combine pulses and grains or wholemeal breads in relatively equal amounts.

- Combine pulses and dairy products (you need less dairy than pulses).

- Combine grains or wholemeal breads and dairy products (you need less dairy than grains).

- Include eggs or (preferably low-fat) dairy products somewhere in your meal (this could be in the form of a pudding).

- Include tofu or other soya products somewhere in your meal.

Here are guidelines for obtaining the minimum of fat (everybody needs a certain amount, but most of us get more than we need) from a vegetarian diet:

- Concentrate on grains, pulses, vegetables, fish, chicken and turkey without the skin and rabbit, which are naturally low in fat.

- Keep cheese, especially hard cheeses, to a minimum.

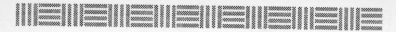

- Use skimmed milk, low-fat yoghurt and low-fat cottage cheese instead of full-fat dairy products. *Read labels*: they usually list the fat content.

- Eliminate butter and cream. Use margarine very sparingly. Cook with vegetable oils and keep them to a minimum.

- Avoid nuts. Snack on crudités and salads instead.

- USE THE RECIPES IN THIS BOOK

How to use this book

This book is divided into a recipe section followed by several menu plans. You may also want to devise your own menus. All the recipes are low in fats, so you can make your own choices. Certainly most people are habitual about breakfast and might want to stick to one or two of the different menus. Remember that this isn't a crash diet; it is a moderately low-calorie diet and, more important, the calories are efficient, useful ones. What this diet *is* is a low-*fat* diet, and fats are what make you fat.

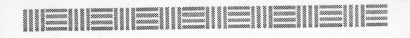

Dining Out

You can stick to this diet even if you tend to dine out a lot. With the exception of fast-food hamburger joints, you can find healthful food in almost every kind of restaurant. Even haute cuisine French restaurants will serve up a simple piece of fish with no sauce or a vegetable plate if you ask. Of course there are many good vegetarian restaurants, but you need not feel restricted to them. Indian and oriental restaurants have a variety of vegetarian dishes (though many Indian restaurants are too heavy-handed with oil for this diet; choose carefully, ordering rice dishes and asking for drier vegetable dishes). Italian restaurants have pastas with tomato sauce or vegetables, salads, vegetable side-dishes and fruit desserts. French restaurants usually have beautiful salads, vegetable side-dishes and eggs, and even a grill will be able to provide you with potatoes and salad.

When you go to a restaurant, look through the entire menu first. Vegetable dishes are usually scattered throughout. I often order two dishes from the entrée section, asking the waiter to bring one of them as a first course and the second as a main dish. If you don't see anything suitable on the menu, ask the waiter if the chef can do something special for you. Especially in better restaurants, chefs are happy to accommodate special diets and often enjoy the challenge.

If you are not a strict vegetarian, order grilled fish, making sure to ask for the fish without butter and with the sauce on the side.

Almost any restaurant will make up a fruit or vegetable plate for you, even if it isn't on the menu. Don't be bashful about asking the waiter; and make sure to tell him not to let the chef pour butter over everything. Ask for a fresh lemon.

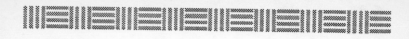

Exercise

The importance of exercise

To lose weight really effectively and keep it off, exercise is essential. This is because sustained physical activity eventually increases your amount of muscle tissue, altering your body chemistry and speeding up your metabolism so that you burn calories more efficiently *even while you sleep.*

Thinness and fatness actually have more to do with the percentage of fat you have than with your actual weight. We all need to have a certain amount of fat, and storage of fat is a natural bodily function. Fat people are just over-proficient at it; they burn calories less easily. But the reason for this is that fat does not require energy. Muscles, on the other hand, do. *Muscles burn calories.* They are full of specific enzymes whose purpose is to burn up calories quickly, and they need lots of calories because movement is our most energy-demanding bodily function. Muscles burn 90 per cent of the calories used up in the body, so the greater your muscle mass, the more calories you will burn all the time. That is, if the muscles are in tone.

That's one reason why crash dieting is self-defeating. When you diet you usually reduce your muscle mass – another reason why you lower your metabolism. Even if you lose pounds, you lose muscle along with the fat, and that does nothing to improve your shape.

Aerobic exercise increases the number of the calorie-burning enzymes located in your muscle cells. It increases the burning of fats and calories throughout the day, not just when you are deliberately exercising. In fact, relatively few calories are burned during the physical activity itself – a good reason for choosing the exercise you like rather than just the one the charts say requires the most energy. It is the cumulative effect that works to transform your body into an independent, self-regulating organism.

When you begin a regular exercise programme you might be surprised and dismayed to find that you are not losing weight. That is, the scales don't look encouraging. In fact you may even gain a few pounds, because muscle is heavier than fat. But soon your shape will begin to change. What you have gained is lean body mass. Exercising reduces the fat stores inside the muscle, making your muscles long, lean and firm. If you rely on dieting alone you will not lose anything but the fat under your skin, and the shape

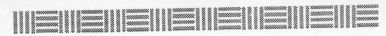

of your body will remain the same. Spot reducing – trying to lose weight from one particular part of your body – doesn't work either, because the calorific demand is small when only one set of muscles is exercised. Spot reducing results simply in a larger muscle with the same fat deposits on top. When large sets of muscles are exercised, fat is drawn from all over the body to meet the muscles' energy requirements. The more muscle you have, the more energy you need to burn, and the more enzymes you have to burn it.

Aerobic exercise

The kind of exercise that results in this overall change in muscle tone and metabolism is *aerobic* exercise. It is steady exercise – uninterrupted for at least 12–20 minutes, depending on the sport – which makes the muscles work hard enough to require lots of oxygen. Regular aerobic exercise – three days a week or more – increases muscle mass so that the body burns more calories at all times.

You should choose an exercise which uses all your muscles fully, and which is not a stop-and-go sport; 15 minutes of jogging is a more effective way of maintaining muscle tone and body weight than 2 hours of tennis (unless you are Martina Navratilova). The activity must be continuous; you can't break it up and exercise twice during the day for 6 minutes each time. And of course, more than 12 minutes will increase your muscle tone and metabolism even further. Devoting extra time does more for you than exercising three days a week for 30 minutes. Certain aerobic exercises require more time to work up to the heart rate necessary for long-term metabolic changes. The benefits will be lost altogether if you exercise *less* than three days a week.

Choosing an aerobic exercise

The most important thing to consider when choosing your form of exercise is: what do you like? If running makes your legs hurt too much, don't run. If you hate getting your hair wet, swimming isn't for you. If you like sociable sports, find a work-out class. Sometimes you won't enjoy sport at first but will grow to love it, because it will make you feel so good.

You must be able to assimilate your activity into your lifestyle. If you

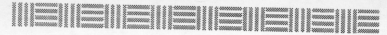

don't have much time then the shortest forms of exercise with the greatest efficiency are the ones to consider. Any exercise may seem like torture at first, if you aren't in shape, but after a while most sports become addictive, and this is the kind of addiction to seek.

No matter what you choose, always begin by doing the minimum and gradually work up to more. Stretch out for 3–5 minutes before and afterwards, to warm up and cool down. Don't push yourself too hard or you may eventually give up.

When you begin to do strenuous exercise, the first 10 minutes are the most excruciating; you get out of breath, and you ache if you are doing aerobics or a jarring sport. But after those 10 minutes you get a second wind and your heart beats comfortably at an elevated rate. Then you can go on for another 10–20 minutes, or longer, and get the maximum out of your exercise.

Here is a list of aerobic exercises to choose from:

walking (20 minutes minimum)

jogging (20 minutes minimum)

cycling (20 minutes minimum)

stationary bicycle (12–15 minutes minimum)

swimming (20 minutes minimum)

skipping rope (12–15 minutes minimum)

aerobic dance (15 minutes minimum)

cross-country skiing (15 minutes minimum)

jumping jacks (12–15 minutes minimum)

rowing (15 minutes minimum)

figure skating (20 minutes minimum)

roller skating (20 minutes minimum)

canoeing and kayaking (15 minutes minimum)

trampolining (15 minutes minimum)

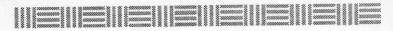

Aerobic and anaerobic exercises and sports

The following activities – called anaerobic – become aerobic in their effect if they involve continuous exertion for at least 20 minutes. For the most part they are stop-and-go exercises and not considered aerobic, but can be excellent for muscle toning and stretching. For the best aerobic bene-fits, supplement them with something from the above list.

Alpine skiing. This can be aerobic if you ski hard enough to raise your heart rate and keep it up for 15 minutes or more. You need long runs for this.

Badminton and volleyball. These can be aerobic if they are power sports, not the kind of Sunday sports that you play on the beach. Usually, though, there is too much starting and stopping for them to be consid-ered aerobic.

Basketball. If you keep moving on the court this can be one of the best aerobic exercises.

Callisthenics. Callisthenics are muscle-toning exercises such as sit-ups, push-ups, leg-lifts and deep kneebends. They are very good for firming the body and making you more flexible, but they are not really aerobic exercises. Some people regard jumping jacks and running on the spot as callisthenics, probably because they are often combined with true callisthenic exercises in work-outs for a marvellous overall effect on the body.

Fencing. This can be aerobic during training, but is a stop-and-go exercise during matches.

Handball and squash. These sports can be highly aerobic if you are well matched with your opponents and have long, strenuous rallies. Handball is less likely to be aerobic than squash and racketball.

Hockey, lacrosse and soccer. These field sports can be aerobic for play-ers in forward positions if activity is constant for over 20 minutes. For full-back positions, and definitely for the goalkeeper, these are stop–start sports.

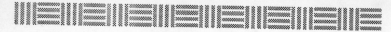

Karate, judo, aikido, kung fu, tae kwon do. These Far Eastern martial arts can be aerobic if your training sessions are intense work-outs, 2 hours long. Beginners would not get aerobic benefit for some time. Matches are stop and go.

Tennis. This can be aerobic if the rallies are long and you hit the ball hard and far, so that you and your opponent run a lot.

Water-skiing. This can be aerobic if you ski steadily and move in and out of the wake a lot.

Non-aerobic short-duration exercise

American-style football

Gymnastics

Isometrics

Sprinting

Track and field sports (except running)

Weightlifting

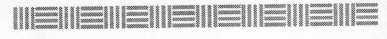

General Techniques and Cooking Instructions

Preparing fruits and vegetables

Apples and pears. To dice or chop, cut straight down each side of the stem, so that there are four pieces and the stem and core are left in one straight-sided centre piece. Then slice each piece in one direction, give it a quarter-turn and cut again.

Broccoli and cauliflower. To break into florets, cut cauliflower in half, cut away the stem and break off the flowers. Cut broccoli tops off the stems and break into smaller flowers.

Cabbage. To shred cabbage, cut into quarters and cut away the thick stem. Then cut each quarter into thin strips, using a long, sharp knife.

Corn on the cob. To remove corn kernels from the cob, stand the cob upright on a plate and run a knife down between the kernels and the cob.

Garlic. First pull off the number of cloves you need from the head. To peel, place the clove on a cutting board and pound it once with the bottom of a jar, or place the flat side of a wide cutting knife over it and lean on the knife. The clove will burst and the skin will pop off. Either put the clove through a garlic press or chop it, holding down the tip of your knife with one hand while you rock the knife up and down with your other hand. Continue with this motion until the clove is as finely chopped as you wish.

Herbs. To chop herbs such as parsley or basil, pick the leaves off the stems, place them on a cutting board and, using a large knife, chop with quick, rapid strokes, holding down the tip of the knife with your spare hand. The herbs will spread out as you chop, but just keep pushing them back to the centre. Alternatively, pick the leaves off the stems, place them in a jar and cut them with scissors. Parsley, but not other herbs, can be chopped in a food processor.

11

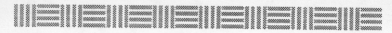

Lettuce and spinach. Washing leafy vegetables can be very tedious, but there's nothing worse than chomping down on sandy lettuce. If you wash a large quantity at a time, you won't have to face the task every time you want a salad. Separate the leaves and fill the sink or a bowl with cold water. Place the lettuce or spinach leaves in the water, take each individual leaf and run it under cold water, rubbing it with your thumbs if necessary to make sure that all the grit is washed off. Soak once more, drain on kitchen towels and pat dry, or dry in a salad spinner (one of the greatest inventions of the modern kitchen). To store, wrap the leaves in towels and place, towel and all, in plastic bags. Seal well and store in the lower part of your refrigerator.

Mushrooms. If the mushrooms are not at all sandy, simply cut off the very ends of the stems and wipe the mushrooms with a damp cloth. If they are sandy, cut away the stem ends, run the mushrooms briefly under cold water and rub off the sand with your thumbs. Wipe dry with a paper towel or cloth and slice thin.

Onions. First cut in half lengthwise – that is, from the stem end to the other end, along one of the lines. Cut off the very ends and remove the skin from each half. (Do this near the sink with the cold water running and you won't cry so much.)

   To slice or cut into strips, lay one half flat-side down on your cutting board and cut across the onion in thin strips, starting at one end and working towards the centre; hold the onion down at the opposite end with your other hand. As the knife nears your fingers, turn the onion half around and, holding on to the side you have already cut to steady the onion, cut again towards the centre. To dice, give the half onion a quarter-turn and cut across the slices at a right-angle.

   To cut rings, do not cut the onion in half but remove the skin from the whole onion by cutting a lengthwise slit through the skin one layer deep, all the way around, then removing the skin. Cut the onion crosswise (across the lines) into rings.

Oranges and grapefruit. To peel and cut away the white pith at the same time, using a very sharp knife cut off the skin in a spiral, starting at the stem end and tilting the knife inwards slightly. Hold the fruit over a bowl, as the juice will drip.

   If you are peeling the fruit just to eat or to divide into sections and

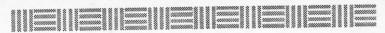

therefore don't need to get rid of the pith, quarter the fruit just through the skin with a sharp knife, then peel off the skin in neat quarters.

Sweet peppers. To cut into strips or dice, cut in half lengthwise (from the stem down) and gently remove the stem, seeds and membranes. Proceed as for onions, cutting into lengthwise strips, then crosswise into dice. For rings, cut off the top from the whole pepper, remove the seeds and membranes, and cut crosswise.

Tomatoes. To peel, bring a pan of water to a rolling boil and drop in the tomatoes. Count to twenty, remove the tomatoes from the water and hold them under cold running water for several seconds. The skin will come away easily.

To seed, cut in half crosswise (halfway between the stem end and the bottom) and squeeze each half over a bowl. Don't worry about crushing the tomato, because you are going to cook it anyway.

To chop tomatoes, cut several strips in one direction across each tomato half, then give the half tomato a quarter-turn and cut across in the other direction.

Slicing several vegetables at once. Long vegetables like carrots, cucumbers and courgettes can be lined up on a cutting board and, with a long, sharp knife, simultaneously cut into crosswise slices. Work deliberately and carefully to avoid cutting yourself.

Cooking dried beans, grains and pasta

Dried beans. With the exception of lentils and split peas, pulses must be soaked for at least 4 hours, and preferably overnight, before you cook them. Wash the beans and pick them over to make sure there are no little pebbles mixed in with them. Use three parts water to one part beans, and if your water is very hard, use bottled water. Drain the water before you cook, and cook in fresh water. For a very tasty dish of beans, sauté one onion and a few cloves of garlic in your cooking pan before adding the beans. When the onion is soft, add the beans and three parts water and bring to a rolling boil. Make sure the volume of the pan is at least one-third greater than that of the beans and water, as they will bubble up fairly dramatically. Reduce the heat, cover the pan and

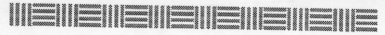

simmer for 1 hour (45 minutes is sufficient cooking for lentils and split peas). Add salt, additional garlic and herbs to taste, and continue to simmer, covered, for another hour, or until soft.

Grains. See pp. 161–3.

Pasta. Bring a large pan of water to a rolling boil. Add salt and a teaspoon of vegetable or safflower oil, then drop in the pasta. Give the pasta a stir with a long-handled spoon so that it doesn't stick together. You want to cook the pasta only until it is cooked through but still firm to the bite – *al dente* – and this will take anything from 4 to 10 minutes, depending on the kind of pasta. Test it after 4 minutes and keep testing every minute until it is done. Drain and proceed with your recipe.

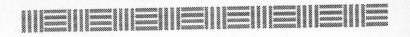

Ingredients

Some of the ingredients in the recipes that follow might be unfamiliar to you, so a short glossary is given below. This is by no means a complete list of grains, legumes, etc.; it includes only those items called for in the recipes in this book.

Grains

Barley. A hearty grain with a chewy texture and nutty taste. Very good in soups.

Brown rice. This is unrefined rice, which has a very nutty, wholesome flavour. Both long and short-grain brown rice are available and are easy to find in supermarkets as well as in wholefood shops. Brown rice takes longer to cook than white, but is worth the wait. It is very high in B vitamins, an excellent source of complex carbohydrates and provides very good protein when eaten in combination with dried beans, dairy products or eggs.

Bulgur. Cracked wheat that has been pre-cooked and dried. It is very quick to prepare: all you have to do is pour on boiling water and let it stand for about 20 minutes. Bulgur has a nutty taste and fluffy texture, and has the same nutritional characteristics as brown rice (see above).

Couscous. Another pre-cooked cracked-wheat product, made from hard, white semolina wheat. It is very light and has a silky texture. All you need to do to prepare it is pour on warm water. It makes a delicious, quick breakfast grain. Couscous is available from imported-food stores and many wholefood shops.

Cracked wheat. This differs from bulgur (see above) in that it hasn't been pre-cooked. It makes a great breakfast cereal.

Kasha. Buckwheat groats — small pyramid-shaped grains from which buckwheat flour is milled. The flavour is distinctive — earthy and nutty — and delicious.

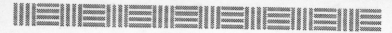

Millet. A delicate, nutty-tasting grain that looks like tiny yellow beads. Substitute it for brown rice whenever you want a change. It also makes a nice breakfast grain, and millet pudding is a fine dessert (see p.205).

Rolled or flaked oats. Porridge oats. High in fibre, these make a terrific breakfast.

Flaked wheat, rye and triticale. All these resemble oat flakes, but they are a little stiffer in texture. Triticale is a hybrid grain made from wheat and rye. All these flakes are made by pressing the whole wheat, rye or triticale berries. Mix them together with oat flakes for granolas and mixed-grain cereals.

Wheatgerm. The embryo of the wheat kernel, these tiny flakes are high in oil, protein and vitamins E and B. Keep wheatgerm refrigerated, as it becomes rancid quickly.

Pulses

Black beans. Black, medium-sized beans with a rich, satisfying flavour. Great for all Mexican dishes.

Black-eyed beans. Medium-sized, oval-shaped, creamy-white beans with a black spot on one side. They have a savoury, warming flavour.

Borlotti beans. These are medium-sized, brown-speckled beans, popular in many Italian dishes. They have a rich texture and a mild flavour.

Chick peas (or garbanzos). Large, round beans with a distinctive, nutty flavour. Great in salads, soups and blended as a spread.

Kidney beans. Fairly large reddish-brown beans, these have a rich, slightly sweet, slightly metallic taste. They are good in salads, soups and chillis.

Lentils. These have a distinctive, satisfying flavour and make a delicious soup or salad. Green lentils are small and dark olive green, with a slightly more peppery flavour than brown lentils. Yellow and red lentils have the mildest flavour. Use green or brown lentils for the recipes in this book unless otherwise instructed.

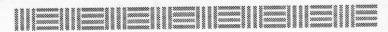

Haricot beans. These have a subtle, elegant flavour and are terrific in soups and salads. They are medium-sized oval beans with a creamy-white colour.

Pinto beans. Medium-sized, speckled, light-brown beans. They are standard in Mexican food. Their flavour is less pronounced than that of either kidney beans or black beans.

Soy beans. These are higher in protein than any of the other legumes. Their protein is complete, and they are very economical. Alone they are not very tasty, but with other beans they are good, and roasted they are superb. Tofu is made from soy beans (see p. 18).

Other essentials

Alfalfa sprouts. Tiny, delicate sprouts formed from alfalfa seeds. Substitute them for lettuce in sandwiches – they don't get soggy; or add them to salads whenever you wish. They are high in protein, vitamins and minerals. They are easy to find in supermarkets as well as in wholefood shops. Other good sprouts are mung-bean sprouts, lentil sprouts and sunflower sprouts.

Arrowroot. This is basically the same as cornflour and is used as a thickener. Like cornflour, it must be dissolved in a little cold liquid before it is used or it will lump.

Dijon mustard. This is French-style mustard with a sharp flavour, not at all sweet. It is essential for many dressings.

Fromage blanc. A fermented dairy product that comes in very low-fat versions. It is like whipped cottage cheese and has a slightly tart flavour. It is available from supermarket dairy sections.

Olive oil. Olive oil contains 'good' cholesterol, the kind that helps lower overall cholesterol. It is a very good oil to use, in moderation, in cooking and for salad dressings.

Safflower and sunflower oil. These oils are very low in polyunsaturates, and if made by a reputable company will not contain added stabilisers. Store in the refrigerator to prevent rancidity (which you can't always taste).

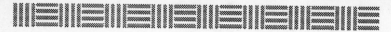

Sesame tahini. This is a butter made from ground sesame seeds. It has a marvellous nutty flavour and is a tasty addition to many tofu dishes and salad dressings.

Tamari soy sauce. A rich, dark soy sauce made by a long, natural fermentation process.

Tofu. This is bean curd, made from soy milk. It is the equivalent of soy cheese. It is a miracle food, very high in protein, low in calories and fat, economical and extremely versatile. By itself it is bland, with a spongy texture; but, like a sponge, it will absorb the flavours of whatever it is cooked with, and as it cooks its texture firms up. It can also be blended into sauces and a low-fat mayonnaise-like vinaigrette, and can be beaten up and baked as a quiche. It must be kept in a bowl of water in the refrigerator. Tofu is available in supermarkets as well as from wholefood shops.

Stocking the larder

The following are items which come up repeatedly in the recipes. Since grains and pulses keep well in tightly sealed jars, you might add your favourite ones to this list so that you will have them around whenever you want them.

Staples

Baking powder
Bicarbonate of soda
Cornflour or arrowroot
Dijon mustard
Dried fruit (such as raisins, prunes, currants, apricots) for
　muffins and fruit butters
Dry white wine
Fresh garlic
Fresh ginger (store in a jar of sherry in the refrigerator)
Fruit preserves (unsweetened; homemade or commercial)
Honey (preferably a light, mild-flavoured kind)
Marmite

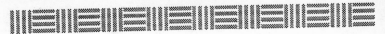

Olive oil
Onions
Safflower or sunflower oil
Sesame oil
Sesame seeds
Sesame tahini
Sherry
Soy sauce
Sunflower seeds
Treacle
Vanilla essence
Vinegar – both cider and wine vinegar
Vegetable *bouillon* cubes

Herbs

Basil
Bay leaves
Caraway seeds
Cayenne (whole and ground)
Dill seeds
Marjoram
Oregano
Paprika
Rosemary
Sage
Tarragon
Thyme

Spices

Allspice
Cardamom
Cayenne
Chilli powder
Cinnamon
Coriander
Cumin seeds
Ground cumin
Curry powder
Dried ginger
Nutmeg
Peppercorns (black)

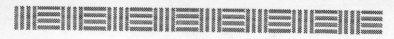

THE RECIPES

Breads and Breakfasts

This section introduces low-fat, high-fibre alternatives to the high-fat, high-cholesterol traditional English breakfast. Eggs are not eliminated here, but instead of 2 whole eggs in a portion of scrambled eggs, for instance, I whole egg and 1 egg white will be used. The most important dishes are the cereals, which provide bulk and will keep you going all morning. You can supplement these with 4fl. oz (120ml) skimmed milk to complement the protein in the cereals. If time is a problem in the morning, you can make porridge in a thermos the night before simply by pouring boiling water over the cereal. Uncooked muesli, however, takes only minutes to prepare and will make a real difference to how you feel throughout the morning.

Breakfast being a meal of habit, you may settle on one or two favourites here and repeat them throughout the week.

Alternatives to butter. Butter isn't the only thing to spread on toast. Even margarine is high in fats, so try these alternatives (a breakfast portion of toast would include 2 slices; a very low-calorie portion is 1 slice):

Fromage blanc (see p. 17): 1 tablespoon per slice

Low-fat Cream Cheese (see p. 24): 1 tablespoon per slice

Prune Butter, Apple Purée or Apricot Purée (see pp. 25 and 195): 1 tablespoon per slice

Cottage cheese: 1 tablespoon per slice

Peanut butter: 2 teaspoons per slice

Beverages. I recommend cutting coffee and tea to a minimum, as caffeine can stimulate the appetite and causes extreme fluctuations in blood sugar. If you take milk in your tea or coffee, substitute skimmed or semi-skimmed milk for whole milk and eliminate sugar. Orange juice and grapefruit juice, freshly squeezed if possible, will provide you with your daily vitamin C requirements. You could also substitute a whole orange or half a grapefruit.

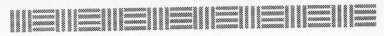

Basic Wholemeal Loaf

2 loaves

2 teaspoons active dried yeast
1¼ pints (750ml) lukewarm water
2 tablespoons mild-flavoured honey, or 1 tablespoon malt extract
2lb (900g) 100 per cent wholemeal flour
2½ teaspoons salt (you can use up to 1 tablespoon if desired)
2 tablespoons sunflower or safflower oil
2–3oz (55–85g) additional wholemeal or unbleached white flour
  for kneading

Optional
1 egg, beaten with 2 tablespoons water, for glaze
2 tablespoons sesame seeds

Dissolve the yeast in the water and let it sit for 5–10 minutes. Stir in the honey or malt extract.

Mix together half the wholemeal flour and the salt. Gradually stir this mixture into the water, a cupful at a time. Use a whisk to obtain a smooth batter. When this portion of the flour has been added, fold in the oil and gradually stir in the remaining 1lb (450g) flour.

As soon as you can, place a generous amount of wholemeal or unbleached white flour on your kneading surface and scrape out the dough. Now begin kneading, using a pastry scraper to facilitate folding the dough, and frequently adding flour to the work surface.

Knead for 15–20 minutes, flouring your hands and the work surface often. The dough will be very sticky at first – you will really need a pastry scraper to turn it, and you will need a lot of flour on your hands – but it will stiffen up after about 5 minutes. At the end of the kneading, the dough will be dense and elastic, though still tacky on the surface. Sprinkle a little more flour on to your work surface and shape the dough into a ball.

Rinse out your bowl and dry it. Lightly oil the bowl and place the dough in it, seam-side up first, then seam-side down. Cover the bowl tightly with clingfilm and a tea-towel. Allow the dough to rise in a warm spot for 1½–2 hours. It should double in bulk and soften considerably during the rising.

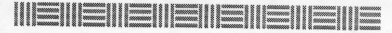

Punch the dough down, cover it and allow it to rise again for 1 hour (this rise can be omitted; the loaves will be slightly denser).

Turn the dough out on to a lightly floured work surface, shape it into a ball and cut it in half. Shape the two halves into balls and let them sit for 10 minutes, so that the dough relaxes.

Now form the loaves. Oil two 8 x 4-inch loaf tins and place the dough in, upside down first, then right-side up. Brush the loaves with glaze, if using, sprinkle with the optional sesame seeds, and brush again with glaze. Cover with a damp tea-towel and set in a warm place to rise for 20–45 minutes if this is the third rising, 45–90 minutes if this is the second rising, until the tops of the loaves curve up above the edges of the tins and the sides reach the tops of the tins.

Meanwhile, pre-heat the oven to 350°F/180°C/gas mark 4. Just before baking, slash the loaves across the top with a razor blade or a sharp knife. Place them in the oven and bake for 50–55 minutes, or until the loaves are a nutty-brown colour and respond to tapping with a hollow sound.

Remove the loaves from the oven and take them out of the tins. (It may be necessary to run a knife between the edge of the tin and the bread.) Cool on racks, laying the bread on its side.

Note This dough will vary, depending on the coarseness of the flour. If the flour is very coarsely ground, you might want to substitute some 85 per cent wholemeal flour for some of the 100 per cent wholemeal – say one quarter of the total flour.

Wholemeal Bagels

1 dozen

For the dough
2 tablespoons active dried yeast
12fl. oz (340ml) lukewarm water
1 tablespoon mild-flavoured honey or malt extract
1 scant tablespoon salt
12oz (340g) wholemeal flour or wholemeal pastry flour
4–6oz (115–170g) unbleached white flour, as needed

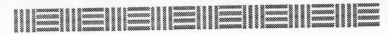

For the boiling
4 pints (2.5 litres) water
1 tablespoon sugar or malt extract

For the topping
1 egg white, beaten with 1 tablespoon water, for glaze
2 tablespoons sesame seeds, poppy seeds, coarse salt,
   finely chopped onion or caraway seeds (these are all optional)

Dissolve the yeast in the lukewarm water in a large bowl, or in the bowl or your electric mixer, stir in the honey or malt extract and let it sit for 10 minutes. Stir in half the wholemeal flour and the salt, and beat vigorously with a whisk or at medium speed (2 on a Kenwood) in a mixer fitted with the mixing attachment for about 5 minutes.

Kneading the bread by hand. Fold in the remaining wholemeal flour. Place 4oz (115g) of the unbleached white flour on your kneading surface and scrape out the dough. Knead, adding more unbleached white flour as necessary, for 10 minutes, until the dough is stiff and elastic. Shape it into a ball.

Using an electric mixer. Add the remaining wholemeal flour and 4oz (115g) of the unbleached white flour. Mix together with the mixing attachment, then change to the dough hook. Mix at low speed (1 on a Kenwood) for 2 minutes, then at medium speed (2 on a Kenwood) for 6–8 minutes. If the dough seems very wet and sticky, sprinkle in up to 2oz (55g) more unbleached white flour. Scrape out the dough on to a lightly floured surface and knead for a minute or so by hand, until the dough is stiff and elastic. Shape it into a ball.

Clean and oil your bowl and place the dough in it, seam-side up first, then seam-side down. Cover the bowl with clingfilm and a tea-towel, and set it in a warm place for the dough to rise for 1½ hours, or until it has doubled in bulk.

Punch down the dough and turn it out on to your work surface. Divide it into twelve equal pieces, shape these into balls and let them rest for 5 minutes, covered lightly with clingfilm.

Meanwhile, combine the 4 pints (2.5 litres) water and the sugar or malt extract and bring to the boil in a large pan over a high heat.

Now shape the bagels. Gently flatten each ball of dough slightly and make a hole in the centre by sticking your thumb through and spreading the centre apart with your fingers. Stretch the hole out so that it's a little

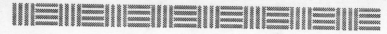

larger than you want it to look when the bagels are done, because as they prove and bake the holes will shrink. Place the bagels on a lightly floured surface and cover them lightly with clingfilm or a tea-towel. Let them rise for 10 minutes.

Pre-heat the oven to 450°F/230°C/gas mark 8.

Now boil the bagels to get the beginning of your sleek, chewy crust. Have the water gently boiling. Using a wide, slotted spatula or a skimmer, gently lift the bagels, in batches of two or three, and lower them into the simmering water. After 30 seconds flip the bagels over so that they boil on both sides. Simmer for 30 seconds more, then carefully lift them from the water with a skimmer or slotted spatula and drain them on a tea-towel. Repeat with the remaining bagels.

Oil a couple of baking sheets and sprinkle them with cornmeal. Gently brush the bagels with the glaze. Sprinkle with the topping of your choice and transfer them to the baking sheets. Bake in the hot oven for 30 minutes, switching the position of the sheets halfway through. Then 10 minutes before the bagels are done, flip them over so that their bottoms won't brown too much. Bagels are done when they are dark brown and shiny.

Remove them from the oven and cool them on a rack.

Low-fat Cream Cheese

8oz (225g)

8oz (225g) low-fat cottage cheese
4 tablespoons natural low-fat yoghurt

Blend together the cottage cheese and yoghurt in a food processor or electric mixer until smooth. Use it as a spread, instead of full-fat cream cheese, on wholemeal bread and bagels.

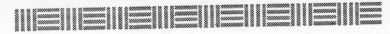

Prune Butter

½ pint (285ml)

This makes a delicious spread for morning toast.

6oz (170g) prunes, stoned
boiling water to cover
4fl. oz (120ml) natural low-fat yoghurt (optional)

Place the prunes in a bowl, pour on boiling water to cover and allow them to sit overnight or for several hours. Drain, retaining a little of the liquid. Purée in a food processor or blender, using a little of the soaking liquid, if necessary, to moisten. Stir in the optional yoghurt. Use as a spread for toast.

Apple Purée or Butter

1 pint (570ml)

2lb (900g) apples, peeled, cored and chopped
4fl. oz (120ml) apple juice

Optional
1 tablespoon mild-flavoured honey
¼–½ teaspoon nutmeg
½–1 teaspoon cinnamon
juice of 1 lemon

Combine all the ingredients in a saucepan and simmer together over a low heat for an hour, stirring from time to time with a wooden spoon, until the mixture is thoroughly softened. If you want a more concentrated purée, continue to cook the mixture to reduce it. Purée in a food processor or blender, or put through a food mill. Cool and transfer to a clean glass jar. Keep in the refrigerator. Use as a spread on toast; or eat as a dessert, served warm or chilled, plain or with yoghurt.

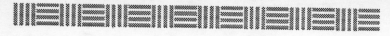

Cornbread or Cornbread Muffins

1 loaf or 12 muffins

6oz (170g) stoneground cornmeal
2oz (55g) wholemeal flour
³/₄ teaspoon salt
1 tablespoon baking powder
¹/₂ teaspoon bicarbonate of soda
8fl. oz (225ml) natural low-fat yoghurt
4fl. oz (120ml) skimmed milk
1 tablespoon mild-flavoured honey
2 eggs
1 tablespoon safflower or sunflower oil
1 tablespoon low-fat margarine

Pre-heat the oven to 425°F/220°C/gas mark 7.

Sift together the cornmeal, wholemeal flour, salt, baking powder and bicarbonate of soda in a bowl. In a separate bowl beat together the yoghurt, milk, honey, eggs and oil.

Place the margarine in a 9 x 9-inch baking tin or a 9-inch cast-iron frying pan and place it in the oven for a few minutes, until the margarine melts and begins to sizzle. Remove from the oven and brush the melted margarine all over the sides and bottom of the tin or pan. Pour any remaining margarine into the liquid mixture.

Fold the wet ingredients into the flour mixture. Do this quickly, without overworking the batter. Don't worry if there are a few lumps. Pour the batter into the prepared baking tin or into prepared muffin tins and bake for 30–35 minutes for a loaf, 20 minutes for muffins, until the top of the bread is brown and a tester comes out clean. Remove from the tin and cool on a rack.

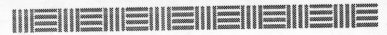

Overnight Bran Muffins

16–20 muffins

You don't have to let this batter sit overnight, but it makes breakfast very easy. The batter will last for a week in the refrigerator, so you could make up a large quantity on Sunday night and have the makings for fresh muffins for every day of the week. The muffins are moist and sweet.

3oz (85g) raisins or sultanas
12fl. oz (340ml) boiling water
6oz (170g) bran
2 eggs
3fl. oz (90ml) sunflower oil
2fl. oz (60ml) mild-flavoured honey
12fl. oz (350ml) buttermilk or skimmed milk, soured with 1 tablespoon
   lemon juice
6oz (170g) wholemeal flour
4oz (115g) unbleached white flour
2½ teaspoons bicarbonate of soda
½ teaspoon salt

Place the raisins or sultanas in a bowl and pour on the boiling water. Allow to sit for 5 minutes, then stir in the bran and allow to sit for another 10 minutes.

Beat together the eggs, oil and the honey. Stir in the buttermilk or sour milk. Stir the raisins and bran, with their liquid, into the milk-and-egg mixture. Combine well.

In a separate bowl, sift together the flours, bicarbonate of soda and salt. Fold this into the liquid mixture. Cover with clingfilm or foil and refrigerate overnight, or bake right away.

When you are ready to bake, pre-heat the oven to 400°F/200°C/gas mark 6 and oil the muffin tins. Give the batter a stir, and spoon it into the tins.

Bake for 20–30 minutes, until the muffins are puffed, brown and cooked through. Remove them from the oven, allow them to cool for 15 minutes (or more) in the tins, then remove them from the tins and cool them on racks.

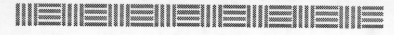

Orange–Apricot Muffins

15–18 muffins

2 oz (55g) dried apricots, chopped
boiling water to cover
2oz (55g) bran
2 oranges
4fl. oz (120ml) skimmed milk
2 eggs
2 tablespoons mild-flavoured honey
2 tablespoons safflower or sunflower oil
4oz (115g) wholemeal flour
3oz (85g) unbleached white flour
2 teaspoons baking powder
½ teaspoon salt

Place the chopped dried apricots in a bowl and pour on boiling water to cover. Let them sit for 10 minutes, while you prepare the batter, then drain the apricots and squeeze them dry between paper towels.

Pre-heat the oven to 375°F/190°C/gas mark 5. Oil or butter the muffin tins.

Squeeze enough juice from the oranges to make 4fl. oz (120ml). Combine this with the milk. Take one of the squeezed orange rinds and chop it coarsely. Place it in a blender with the milk, eggs, honey and oil, and blend until the rind is finely chopped.

Sift together the dry ingredients. Add the wet ingredients and quickly mix together. Fold in the chopped apricots.

Spoon the batter into the prepared muffin tins and bake for 20 minutes, or until the muffins are lightly browned and a tester comes out clean. Cool the muffins in the tins, then remove them and serve, or store them in plastic bags. These can be frozen.

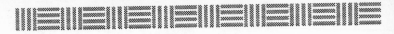

Banana–Nut Muffins or Bread

16 muffins or 1 loaf

These are moist, chewy and dense. The batter is quite thick.

8oz (225g) wholemeal flour or wholemeal pastry flour
1/2 teaspoon bicarbonate of soda
2 teaspoons baking powder
1/2 teaspoon salt
1 teaspoon cinnamon
1/2 teaspoon nutmeg
4 tablespoons safflower or sunflower oil
4 tablespoons mild-flavoured honey
1 teaspoon vanilla essence
2 eggs
3 medium-sized ripe bananas, mashed
4fl. oz (120ml) natural low-fat yoghurt
2oz (55g) sunflower seeds or chopped walnuts

Pre-heat the oven to 375°F/190°C/gas mark 5. Butter muffin tins or a loaf tin.

Sift together the flours, bicarbonate of soda, baking powder, salt and spices.

Beat together the oil, honey, vanilla essence and eggs. Stir in the banana and yoghurt.

Quickly stir the wet ingredients into the dry, along with the nuts. Spoon the batter into the muffin tins or loaf tin. Bake the muffins for 15–20 minutes and bread for 50 minutes, until a tester comes out clean. Cool in the tins for 20 minutes, then remove. These can be frozen.

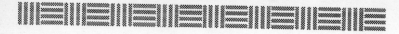

Apple–Raisin Muffins

15 muffins

4oz (115g) wholemeal flour
2 teaspoons baking powder
½ teaspoon salt
1 teaspoon ground cinnamon
½ teaspoon allspice
4oz (115g) bran
2 eggs
4 tablespoons safflower or sunflower oil
4 tablespoons mild-flavoured honey
1 teaspoon vanilla essence
8fl. oz (225ml) skimmed milk or natural low-fat yoghurt
1 apple, peeled, cored and chopped
4 tablespoons raisins

Pre-heat the oven to 375°F/190°C/gas mark 5. Lightly butter muffin tins.
    Sift together the flour, baking powder, salt and spices. Stir in the bran.
    Beat together the eggs, oil, honey, vanilla essence and milk or yoghurt.
Quickly stir the liquid ingredients into the dry and combine well. Fold in
the apple and raisins.
    Spoon the batter into the muffin tins and bake for 20 minutes. Cool for
10 minutes or longer in the tins, then remove the muffins from the tins
and serve them hot or cooled. These can be frozen.

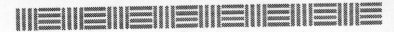

Blueberry–Rice Muffins

15 muffins

5oz (140g) wholemeal flour
2 teaspoons baking powder
½ teaspoon salt
3 tablespoons mild-flavoured honey
4 tablespoons safflower or sunflower oil
I egg
6fl. oz (180ml) skimmed milk or natural low-fat yoghurt
5oz (140g) blueberries
6oz (170g) cooked brown rice (other grains, such as bulgur,
  cracked wheat, millet or barley may be substituted)

Pre-heat the oven to 400°F/200°C/gas mark 6. Lightly butter the muffin tins.
  Sift together the flour, baking powder and salt.
  Beat together the honey, oil, egg and milk. Stir the liquid ingredients into the dry. Fold in the blueberries and brown rice or other cooked grains.
  Spoon the batter into the prepared muffin tins and bake for 20 minutes. Cool for 10 minutes in the tins, then remove the muffins from the tins and serve them warm or cooled. These can be frozen.

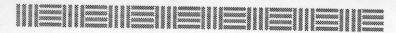

Cranberry Muffins

14 muffins

3oz (85g) wholemeal flour
3oz (85g) rye flour
3oz (85g) stoneground yellow cornmeal
2 teaspoons baking powder
1/4 teaspoon salt
1oz (30g) bran
2 eggs
4 tablespoons safflower or sunflower oil
2 tablespoons mild-flavoured honey
1/2 pint (285ml) buttermilk
6oz (170g) cranberries, coarsely chopped

Pre-heat the oven to 400°F/200°C/gas mark 6. Lightly butter the muffin tins.

Sift together the flours, cornmeal, baking powder and salt. Stir in the bran.

Beat together the eggs, oil, honey and buttermilk. Stir in the chopped cranberries. Quickly stir the liquid ingredients into the dry.

Spoon the batter into muffin tins and bake for 20–25 minutes. Cool the muffins for 10 minutes or longer in the tins, then remove them from the tins and cool them on racks. These can be frozen.

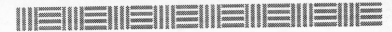

Sweet Potato Muffins

16–18 muffins

4oz (115g) unbleached white flour
4oz (115g) wholemeal pastry flour
2 teaspoons baking powder
1/2 teaspoon bicarbonate of soda
1 teaspoon cinnamon
1/4 teaspoon nutmeg
1/4 teaspoon salt
4 tablespoons safflower or sunflower oil
4 tablespoons mild-flavoured honey
1 egg
3/4lb (340g) cooked mashed sweet potatoes or yams
4fl. oz (120ml) skimmed milk or natural low-fat yoghurt

Pre-heat the oven to 400°F/200°C/gas mark 6. Lightly butter the muffin tins.

Sift together the flours, baking powder, bicarbonate of soda, spices and salt.

Beat together the oil, honey, egg, sweet potatoes or yams and milk or yoghurt. Stir this mixture into the dry ingredients.

Spoon the batter into the prepared muffin tins and bake for 25–30 minutes until the muffins begin to brown. Cool them completely in the tins, then remove; or cool them for 10 minutes in the tins, remove and serve still warm. These can be frozen.

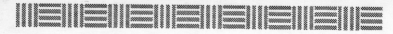

Fruity Oatmeal

serves 4

¾ pint (425ml) water
¾ pint (425ml) skimmed milk
I teaspoon vanilla essence
8oz (225g) flaked oats
¼ teaspoon salt (optional)
3 tablespoons raisins
½–I teaspoon cinnamon
½ teaspoon nutmeg
2 apples, chopped

Combine the water, milk and vanilla essence in a large saucepan (it should be at least 2½-pint (1.5-litre) capacity to avoid boiling over) and bring to a boil. Slowly pour in the flaked oats, stirring all the while with a wooden spoon. Add the salt, raisins, cinnamon, nutmeg and apple, cover and reduce the heat. Simmer over a very low heat for 15–20 minutes, until the liquid is absorbed. Serve at once.

To make the night before

If you are always too rushed in the morning to have a decent breakfast, here is the answer. Before going to bed, place the flaked oats, fruit and spices in a wide-mouthed thermos. Bring the water and milk to a boil, pour them in to the thermos and seal the thermos tightly. In the morning your breakfast will be ready. If it isn't hot enough, simply heat it in a saucepan with a little more water or milk.

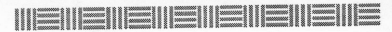

Mixed-grains Porridge

Mix these grains together and keep them on hand for hearty hot cereal.

4oz (115g) flaked oats
6oz (170g) cracked wheat
2oz (55g) cracked millet (this can be done in a blender)
4oz (115g) flaked wheat, rye or triticale
2oz (55g) cornmeal

Store in a tightly sealed jar.

Hot Mixed-grains Porridge with Fruit

serves 4

2 pints (1.2 litres) water, or use half water, half milk
8oz (225g) Mixed-grains Porridge (see above)
4 tablespoons raisins
2 apples, pears or bananas, chopped
1 teaspoon cinnamon
1 teaspoon vanilla essence
1 tablespoon mild-flavoured honey (optional)
salt, to taste

Bring the water or water and milk to a boil and slowly add the porridge mixture, stirring all the while with a wooden spoon. Add the raisins, chopped fruit, cinnamon, vanilla essence, honey and salt, cover and reduce the heat to very low. Simmer for 15–20 minutes. Remove from the heat and serve, topping with skimmed milk or yoghurt if you wish.

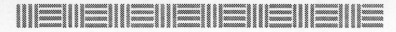

Couscous with Fruit

serves 4

6oz (170g) couscous
3/4 pint (425ml) water
4fl. oz (120ml) apple juice
2 teaspoons vanilla essence
3 tablespoons raisins or sultanas
1 pear, cored and chopped
1 apple, cored and chopped
1/2–1 teaspoon ground cinnamon, to taste
1/2 teaspoon ground nutmeg
1/4 teaspoon allspice
4fl. oz (120ml) natural low-fat yoghurt for topping

Place the couscous in a bowl and pour on the water, which should be warm but not boiling.

Heat the apple juice in a skillet and add the vanilla essence, raisins or sultanas, apple and pear. Cook over a medium heat until the fruit begins to soften: about 3 minutes. Add the spices and cook for another 3–5 minutes.

After about 10 minutes' soaking the couscous should be soft. Add it to the fruits and toss over a medium heat in the pan until heated through. Serve, topping each serving with a generous spoonful of natural low-fat yoghurt if you wish.

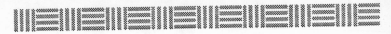

Buckwheat Pancakes

18 pancakes

2 eggs, separated
1 tablespoon mild-flavoured honey
8fl. oz (225ml) skimmed milk
1 tablespoon sunflower or safflower oil
3oz (85g) sifted wholemeal pastry flour
3oz (85g) sifted buckwheat flour
1/4 teaspoon salt
1 teaspoon baking powder
6 tablespoons natural low-fat yoghurt or cottage cheese, for topping

Beat together the egg yolks, honey, milk and oil.

Sift together the flours, salt and baking powder. Stir these into the liquid ingredients.

Beat the egg whites until stiff but not dry. Gently fold them into the batter.

Heat a griddle or a large, heavy, preferably non-stick frying pan over a medium–high heat and brush it with a small amount of oil or butter. Drop the batter on by heaped tablespoonfuls, or small ladlefuls, so that the pancakes are not too big. Cook on the first side until bubbles break through, then turn and cook until golden brown on the other side. Serve at once, topped with one of the fruit purées on pp. 25 and 195 and natural low-fat yoghurt or cottage cheese.

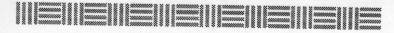

Cottage Cheese–Apple Pancakes

serves 4

4 eggs
4fl. oz (120ml) skimmed milk
8oz (225g) low-fat cottage cheese
1/2 teaspoon vanilla essence
1 tablespoon mild-flavoured honey
2oz (55g) wholemeal flour
1oz (30g) wheatgerm
1 teaspoon cinnamon (or more, to taste)
1 medium-sized apple, chopped
2 teaspoons safflower or sunflower oil, for the griddle or frying pan

Blend together the eggs, milk, cottage cheese, vanilla essence and honey in a blender or food processor.

Stir together the flour, wheatgerm and cinnamon. Stir this into the wet mixture. Stir in the apple.

Heat a heavy, well-seasoned griddle or non-stick frying pan over a medium–high heat. Brush with oil and drop the batter in by heaped spoonfuls (about 3 tablespoons per pancake; using a ladle makes this easier). The griddle or pan must be very hot. Cook on one side until bubbles break through, then carefully turn and cook on the other side until brown. Keep the cooked pancakes warm in a low oven.

Serve topped with natural low-fat yoghurt or Apple Purée (see p. 25).

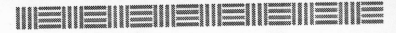

Oatmeal Pancakes

serves 4

3oz (85g) flaked oats
boiling water to cover
8fl. oz (225ml) skimmed milk
1 tablespoon safflower or sunflower oil
2 eggs
1 tablespoon mild-flavoured honey
1/2 teaspoon vanilla essence
a pinch of salt
3oz (85g) wholemeal flour
1 teaspoon baking powder
2 teaspoons safflower or sunflower oil, for the griddle or frying pan

Place the flaked oats in a bowl and pour on just enough boiling water to cover. Let them sit for 10 minutes.

Beat together the milk, oil, eggs, honey and vanilla essence. Stir in the oats. Mix together the salt, flour and baking powder and stir into the wet ingredients. Combine well.

Heat a heavy, well-seasoned griddle or non-stick frying pan over a medium–high heat and brush with oil. Drop the pancakes on by heaped spoonfuls (about 3 tablespoons per pancake). The griddle or pan should be hot. Cook on one side until bubbles break through. Turn and cook on the other side until brown. Keep the cooked pancakes warm in a low oven.

Serve, topping with natural low-fat yoghurt and Apple Purée (see p. 25). These pancakes can be reheated in a medium oven, and will have a satisfying, crisp texture.

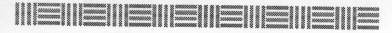

Wholemeal Buttermilk Waffles

serves 4–6

¾ pint (425ml) buttermilk
2 eggs, separated
I tablespoon mild-flavoured honey
I tablespoon safflower or sunflower oil
8oz (225g) wholemeal flour or wholemeal pastry flour
2 teaspoons baking powder
¼ teaspoon salt

Optional

I banana, sliced; or 4oz (115g) blueberries or strawberries; or I apple,
pear or peach, chopped

Blend together the buttermilk, egg yolks, honey and oil in a food processor or electric mixer. Add the flour, baking powder and salt, and combine
well, but don't over-beat. Beat the egg whites until stiff but not dry, and
fold them into the batter. Stir in the optional fruit.

Heat your waffle iron until the indicator shows that it is ready for use.
Fill with batter to about two-thirds full and cook until the iron stops
steaming (about 5 minutes). Waffles should be golden and crisp.

Serve with Prune Butter, Apple Purée, Apricot Purée (see pp. 25 and
195) or blended fruit, and natural low-fat yoghurt.

Note These waffles can be frozen and reheated in a toaster or warm oven.

Scrambled Eggs

serves 4

4 whole eggs
4 egg whites
a pinch of salt
freshly ground pepper, to taste
I teaspoon butter

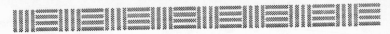

Beat together the whole eggs and the egg whites. Add a pinch of salt and freshly ground pepper, to taste.

Melt the butter in a non-stick frying pan over a low heat. Add the eggs and stir until they reach the desired consistency. Serve at once, with wholemeal toast.

Apple Omelette

serves 4

1 teaspoon safflower oil or low-fat margarine
2 tart apples, such as Granny Smith, cored and sliced
4 eggs
4 egg whites
1/4 teaspoon ground ginger (optional)
2 tablespoons grated Gruyère or Cheddar cheese

Pre-heat the grill.

Heat the oil or margarine in a large, non-stick frying pan and sauté the apples over a medium heat until just tender: about 5 minutes. Spread them evenly over the bottom of the pan.

Beat together the eggs, egg whites and optional ginger in a bowl. Heat the pan over a medium–high heat and pour in the eggs. Shake gently over the heat, and lift the edges of the omelette, tilting the pan so that the eggs will run underneath. When the omelette is almost cooked through (after about 3 minutes) and there is still a runny layer on the top, sprinkle with the grated cheese and place the pan under the grill. Cook under the grill for 2–3 minutes, watching closely, or until the top browns slightly. Remove from the heat and serve, cutting the flat omelette into wedges.

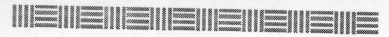

Low-fat Blender Drinks

These make nutritious, low-calorie breakfasts or snacks.

Banana Smoothie

1 serving

1 medium-sized ripe banana
8fl. oz (225ml) natural low-fat yoghurt or skimmed milk
1/2 teaspoon vanilla essence
nutmeg, to taste
2–3 ice cubes

Blend together all the ingredients in a blender until smooth and frothy.

Banana–Peanut Butter Smoothie

1 serving

Add 1 tablespoon peanut butter to the recipe above.

Carob Frappé

1 serving

8fl. oz (225ml) skimmed milk
1 tablespoon carob powder
1 teaspoon vanilla essence
1 teaspoon black treacle
3 ice cubes

Blend together all the ingredients in a blender until smooth and frothy.

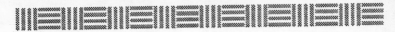

Carob–Banana Frappé

I serving

Add ½ banana (or ½ frozen banana) to the recipe above.

Banana–Strawberry Smoothie

I serving

8fl. oz (225ml) skimmed milk or natural low-fat yoghurt; or 4fl. oz (120ml)
    orange juice and 4fl. oz (120ml) skimmed milk or natural low-fat
    yoghurt
5oz (140g) hulled strawberries, fresh or frozen
½ medium-sized ripe banana
½ teaspoon vanilla essence
nutmeg or cinnamon, to taste (optional)
3 ice cubes

Blend together all the ingredients in a blender until smooth and frothy.

Pineapple–Banana–Mint Smoothie

I serving

4fl. oz (120ml) orange juice
4fl. oz (120ml) natural low-fat yoghurt
½ medium-sized ripe banana
5oz (140g) fresh ripe pineapple, chopped
I tablespoon chopped fresh mint
3 ice cubes

Blend together all the ingredients in a blender until smooth and frothy.

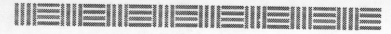

Fruit and Alfalfa Sprout Smoothie

1 serving

8fl. oz (225ml) orange or apple juice
4fl. oz (120ml) natural low-fat yoghurt
2 tablespoons fresh mint
1/2 medium-sized ripe banana
1oz (30g) alfalfa sprouts
3 ice cubes

Blend together all the ingredients in a blender until smooth and frothy.

Carrot–Apple Drink

1 serving

4fl. oz (120ml) natural low-fat yoghurt
1 large carrot, chopped
1 tablespoon wheatgerm or granola
4fl. oz (120ml) apple or orange juice
1/2 teaspoon cinnamon
1/2 apple, cored and chopped
2 figs or stoned prunes
3 ice cubes

Blend together all the ingredients in a blender until smooth and frothy.

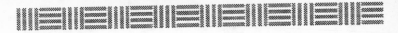

Apple Smoothie

I serving

8fl. oz (225ml) natural low-fat yoghurt, or 4fl. oz (120ml) apple juice
  and 4fl. oz (120ml) natural low-fat yoghurt
1 apple, peeled, cored and chopped
$^1/_2$ teaspoon cinnamon
$^1/_4$ teaspoon nutmeg
$^1/_2$ teaspoon vanilla essence
$^1/_2$ medium-sized ripe banana
$^1/_2$ teaspoon mild-flavoured honey
3 ice cubes

Blend together all the ingredients in a blender until smooth and frothy.

Peach Buttermilk Smoothie

I serving

8fl. oz (225ml) buttermilk
2 fresh ripe peaches, stoned
$^1/_2$ medium-sized ripe banana
1 teaspoon vanilla essence
$^1/_4$ teaspoon cinnamon
nutmeg, to taste
3 ice cubes

Blend together all the ingredients in a blender until smooth and frothy.

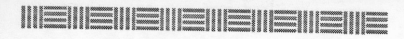

Spreads and Sandwiches

Sandwiches on wholemeal breads can be filling and satisfying at lunchtime, and make nice light suppers as well. But these sandwiches aren't smothered with mayonnaise and stuffed with cheese and/or sandwich meats. Delicious low-fat spreads, pittas filled with pungent Marinated Vegetables or Warm Vegetable Salad, savoury 'Pizza' Sandwiches toasted under the grill – these are just some of the recipes you'll find here (see pp. 49–50)

If you want to cut your calorific intake even further, make open-faced sandwiches using only one slice of bread. Pile the filling high on the bread and cut the *tartine* into small pieces that are easy to handle.

Salads and leftover beans make wonderful fillings for pitta breads, and the pittas are easy to wrap and transport. Use leftovers from last night's dinner. Once you get going you'll never run out of ideas.

Haricot Bean Spread

1¼ pints (750ml)

2 tins haricot beans, drained
2 large cloves garlic
juice of 1 lemon (or more, to taste)
salt and freshly ground pepper, to taste
½–1 teaspoon ground cumin (optional)
1 teaspoon Dijon mustard (or more, to taste – optional)

Purée together all the ingredients in a blender or food processor until smooth. Transfer to a serving dish or covered container and chill. Serve on bread or with crudités.

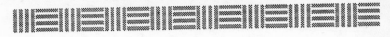

Smoky Aubergine Purée

about ³/₄ pint (425ml)

2¹/₂ lb (1.25kg) aubergine
1¹/₂ teaspoons olive oil
3 tablespoons natural low-fat yoghurt
4 tablespoons lemon juice (or more, to taste)
1–2 cloves garlic, finely chopped or put through a press
salt and freshly ground pepper, to taste
¹/₄ teaspoon ground cumin
2 tablespoons finely chopped parsley
crudités and/or bread or pitta, for serving

Pre-heat the grill. Put the aubergines on an oiled baking sheet and place about 4 inches under the grill. Turn every 5 minutes or so, and grill until the aubergines are charred and soft. Remove them from the heat and allow to cool.

Remove all the charred skin from the aubergines, and carefully squeeze out the liquid. Purée the flesh with the olive oil, yoghurt, lemon juice, garlic, salt, pepper and cumin until smooth, using a food processor, blender or mortar and pestle. Taste and adjust seasonings, then transfer to an attractive serving bowl. Cover and refrigerate, preferably overnight or for several hours.

Shortly before serving, remove the purée from the refrigerator and sprinkle on the parsley. Garnish with crudités, such as thickly sliced red and green peppers, fennel sticks, carrots and cucumbers, and crackers, pitta or thinly sliced bread, and serve.

Vegan version
Omit the yoghurt. Substitute 1 tablespoon sesame tahini.

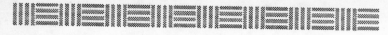

Cucumber–Cottage Cheese Spread
1lb (450g)

12oz (340g) natural low-fat cottage cheese
3oz (85g) cucumber, finely chopped
1 tablespoon chopped fresh dill or parsley
1 teaspoon dill seeds or cumin seeds (optional)
juice of 1/2 lemon
freshly ground pepper, to taste

Combine all the ingredients and mix thoroughly. Use as a spread for sandwiches on wholemeal bread or as a filling for wholemeal pitta breads, or eat as a salad.

Humous
serves 10–12

1/2lb (225g) uncooked chick peas, cooked (see p. 16 for instructions), or a 14oz (395g) tin, drained
2 large cloves garlic
4–6 tablespoons lemon juice, to taste
1/4–1/2 teaspoon ground cumin, to taste
6–8 tablespoons natural low-fat yoghurt
2 tablespoons sesame tahini
salt, to taste

Purée together all the ingredients in a food processor or blender until smooth. Refrigerate in a covered container. Use as a spread on wholemeal bread or pitta bread, or as a dip for vegetables. This will keep for 5 days in the refrigerator.

Vegan version
Substitute cooking liquid from the beans for the yoghurt.

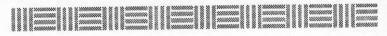

Pizza Sandwiches

When you want something like a pizza, but don't feel like going through the hassle of making the crust, use wholemeal bread. Spread with tomato sauce and the toppings of your choice, top with another piece of bread, wrap in aluminum foil and heat in the oven, or leave open-faced and heat under the grill without wrapping.

Peanut Butter and Honey Tartine

For each tartine

1 tablespoon unsalted, natural peanut butter (no stabilisers, sugar
  or fats added)
1 teaspoon mild-flavoured honey
1 slice wholemeal bread

Spread the peanut butter on the bread and top with honey. This will really get you through the afternoon. It makes a good breakfast too.

Vegetable Pitta Pockets

serves 4

4 wholemeal pitta breads, cut in half
mustard for the bread (optional)
$1/2$ recipe Marinated Vegetables (see p. 59)
1oz (30g) freshly grated Parmesan cheese or Gruyère

Cut the pittas in half and open up the pockets. Spread with mustard if desired. Toss together the vegetables and cheese, and stuff the pockets with the mixture. If not eating right away, wrap tightly in clingfilm and refrigerate.

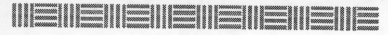

Tofu Salad Sandwich

Use the recipe for Tofu Salad on p. 61. Make sandwiches on wholemeal or granary bread, or fill wholemeal pittas with the mixture.

Spinach and Tofu Pitta Sandwiches

serves 4–6

6oz (170g) spinach, washed, stemmed and dried
10oz (285g) tofu
1–2 teaspoons soy sauce, to taste
8fl. oz (225ml) Tofu Dressing (see p. 54)
4–6 large wholemeal pitta breads, cut in half
1oz (30g) alfalfa sprouts (optional)
sliced tomatoes (optional)

Place the spinach, tofu, soy sauce and dressing in a food processor and chop and blend together, using the pulse action of your processor. The spinach should be finely chopped but not puréed. Stuff the pitta pouches with this mixture, and add sliced tomatoes and alfalfa sprouts if you wish.

Warm Vegetable Salad Sandwiches or Pitta Pockets

Use the recipe for Warm Vegetable Salad on p. 64 (or leftovers from the recipe). Use about 2oz (55g) per sandwich, or 3oz (85g) for pitta pockets, and top with 1 tablespoon grated Gruyère or Cheddar cheese. For a delicious, hot open-faced sandwich, top wholemeal bread with the mixture and 1 tablespoon grated cheese, and put under the grill until the cheese melts.

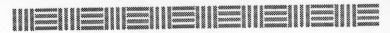

Tuna Salad Pitta Pockets

serves 2

a 5oz (145g) tin tuna fish in brine
3oz (85g) chopped green pepper, or cucumber, or celery
juice of 1 lemon
1 clove garlic, finely chopped or put through a press
1/2–1 teaspoon Dijon mustard, to taste
4–6 tablespoons natural low-fat yoghurt, to taste
2oz (55g) lettuce or alfalfa sprouts
2 wholemeal pitta breads

Drain the tuna fish and mix it with the chopped vegetables, the lemon juice, garlic, mustard and yoghurt. Cut a slit in the end of each pitta bread and line it with lettuce leaves or alfalfa sprouts, then stuff with the tuna mixture. Serve, or wrap in clingfilm and refrigerate until ready to eat.

'Chilidogs'

serves 4

I don't know if 'chilidogs' exist in the UK, but they are very popular in America. Hotdog vendors in Manhattan sell them, and all over the city people can be seen wolfing them down for lunch. A chilidog consists of a hotdog topped with chilli – not exactly low-fat. This tasty version, however, is very healthy indeed.

4 wholemeal hamburger or hotdog buns (available in wholefood
    stores), or wholemeal baps
3/4 pint (450ml) Meatless Chilli (see p. 158)
1oz (30g) Cheddar cheese, grated
shredded lettuce or alfalfa sprouts

Top each bun with Meatless Chilli, a tablespoon of grated cheese, and shredded lettuce or alfalfa sprouts to taste. These tend to drip, so eat them carefully.

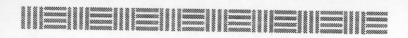

Salads, Dressings and Condiments

I practically live on salads. They become a vehicle for all the beautiful fresh vegetables I find in the market, as well as for many leftovers, especially grains and pulses (see Bulgur Pilaf Salad, p. 72).

There are plenty of substantial salads to choose from here – bean salads like the Lentil Salad on p. 70, or Warm Chick-pea Salad on p. 74; salads made from grains, like the Curried Brown Rice Salad on p. 69 or the Tabouli on p. 73. Potato salad is also filling, and the tofu and egg salads here are very high in protein (as are the bean salads). These can easily serve as main dishes.

More delicate combinations, which would make nice starters, light lunches or side-dishes, are also plentiful here. Among my favourites are the Watercress and Mushroom Salad on p. 67, the Spinach and Tangerine Salad on p. 58 and the Grated Carrot Salad on p. 65.

Some of these salads can also double as sandwich fillings or toppings. One of my favourite lunches is a Tofu Salad Sandwich (p. 50), and I love filling pittas with Marinated Vegetables (p. 59).

The dressings here are low in fat. I have taken traditional vinaigrettes and substituted yoghurt, stock or *bouillon* or tomato juice for the oil, with very good results. I have made a mayonnaise with tofu and a rich green dressing with yoghurt and herbs. Salsa (p. 55), the spicy combination of tomatoes, chillis and fresh coriander that goes so well with Mexican food, also makes a nice dressing. Whatever your tastes, there are plenty of choices here.

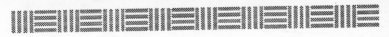

Low-fat Salad Dressings

Low-fat Yoghurt Dressing

approx 1/2 pint (285ml)

juice of 1/2 large lemon
3 tablespoons wine or cider vinegar
I teaspoon Dijon mustard (or more, to taste)
I clove garlic, finely chopped or put through a press (optional)
1/4 teaspoon dried tarragon
freshly ground pepper, to taste
6–8fl. oz (170–225ml) natural low-fat yoghurt, to taste

Mix together the lemon juice, vinegar, mustard, garlic, tarragon and pepper. Whisk in the yoghurt and mix well. Keep in a covered container in the refrigerator for up to a week.

Curried Low-fat Dressing

Use the recipe above, omitting the herbs. Add 1/2 teaspoon ground cumin and 1/2 teaspoon curry powder.

Tomato Dressing

Use the recipe for Low-fat Yoghurt Dressing (above), but substitute either I ripe tomato or 6–8fl. oz (170–225ml) tomato juice for the yoghurt. Blend together all the ingredients in a blender. This is suitable for vegans.

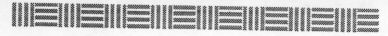

Tofu Dressing

approx. ½ pint (285ml)

juice of 1 lemon
2 tablespoons wine or cider vinegar
4fl. oz (120ml) natural low-fat yoghurt
1 small clove garlic
1 teaspoon Dijon mustard (or more, to taste)
1 teaspoon soy sauce
4oz (115g) tofu
freshly ground pepper, to taste

Place all the ingredients in a blender or food processor and blend together until completely smooth.

Low-fat Green Dressing

12fl. oz (350ml)

To either the Tofu Dressing (above) or the Low-fat Yoghurt Dressing (p. 53) add ½oz (15g) chopped parsley or spinach, washed and dried. Blend together all the ingredients in a food processor or blender until completely smooth.

Low-fat Vegan Dressing

Substitute your choice of the following ingredients for the yoghurt in the above recipes:

vegetable stock or *bouillon* (see p. 80)

cooking liquid from beans

tomato juice

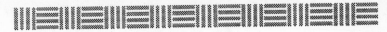

Salsa Fresca

³/₄ pint (425ml)

This is great with Mexican food, but also as a condiment for vegetables.

4 large ripe tomatoes, chopped
¹/₂ small onion, finely chopped
4 tablespoons chopped fresh coriander
2 hot green chilli peppers (or more, to taste), finely chopped
1 tablespoon red wine vinegar
salt, to taste

Mix together all the ingredients in a bowl. Chill until ready to serve. This will keep for 2–3 days in the refrigerator.

Tossed Mixed Green Salad

serves 4–6

³/₄lb (340g) lettuce (any kind), washed well and dried
¹/₂ cucumber, sliced thin
4 radishes, trimmed and sliced thin
4 mushrooms, cleaned, dried and sliced thin
3 spring onions, sliced (optional)
1–2oz (30–55g) beansprouts (optional)
2 tomatoes, cut into wedges
¹/₂ green or red pepper, cut into strips
low-fat dressing of your choice (see pp. 53–4)

Optional
cooked chick peas or beans
cubed tofu
leftover cooked grains, such as rice, bulgur, wheatberries
leftover or freshly steamed vegetables, such as cauliflower, broccoli,
    courgettes, beetroot, green beans, corn, peas

Toss together all the ingredients with the dressing of your choice and serve at once.

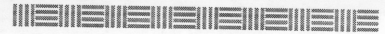

Salade Niçoise

serves 4–6

This salad can be a filling, nutritious meal. In my low-fat version I use water-packed tuna and substitute plain low-fat yoghurt for some of the olive oil in a traditional vinaigrette.

For the vinaigrette

2–3 teaspoons red wine vinegar, to taste
2 tablespoons fresh lemon juice
1 clove garlic, finely chopped or put through a press
1 tablespoon Dijon mustard
2 tablespoons chopped fresh herbs, such as basil, parsley, sage, tarragon, thyme
salt and freshly ground pepper, to taste
2 tablespoons olive oil
6 tablespoons plain low-fat yoghurt

For the salad

4 medium-sized new potatoes, peel scrubbed and left on, diced
1 small head Boston lettuce, leaves separated and washed, then broken into medium to large pieces
½lb (225g) carrots, peeled and grated
1lb (450g) tomatoes, sliced
2 eggs, hard-boiled, peeled and sliced
½lb (225g) green beans, steamed until crisp-tender
1 small cucumber, peeled, seeded and thinly sliced
1 green or red pepper, thinly sliced
1 can water-packed tuna

Prepare the vinaigrette. Combine the vinegar, lemon juice, garlic, mustard, herbs, salt and pepper, and whisk in the olive oil and yoghurt.

Steam or boil the potatoes until tender and toss with the vinaigrette in a large salad bowl. Prepare the remaining vegetables and eggs, add to the bowl, crumble in the tuna fish and toss together. Adjust seasonings and serve.

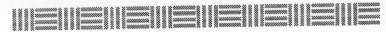

Roasted Sweet Red Peppers

serves 4–6

One of my favourite Mediterranean dishes. This is good to have on hand and will keep for days in the refrigerator.

4–6 medium-sized sweet red peppers
2 large cloves garlic, finely chopped or put through a press
2 tablespoons red wine vinegar (or more to taste)
1 tablespoon olive oil
salt to taste
1–2 tablespoons chopped fresh herbs, if available, such as basil, tarragon,
    parsley, thyme, rosemary

There are several ways to roast the peppers. You can place them directly in a gas flame or under a grill. Or you can place them in a dry frying pan over an electric or gas burner, or in a baking dish in a hot oven. You want all the skin to blister and blacken. Keep turning the peppers until they are uniformly charred, then place in a plastic bag or wrap in a kitchen towel until cool enough to handle.

Peel off the blackened skin, split in half and remove the seeds and inner membranes. Rinse quickly under cool water and pat dry. Cut the halved peppers in half lengthwise, or in wide strips. Place in a bowl or serving dish and toss with the garlic, vinegar, olive oil and salt to taste. Cover and refrigerate until ready to serve. Toss with the fresh herbs shortly before serving.

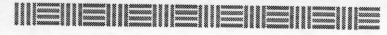

Spinach Salad

serves 4–6

¹/₂lb (225g) fresh spinach, stems removed, washed carefully and dried
4–6 mushrooms, cleaned, stems trimmed and sliced
2 spring onions, sliced (optional)
2 tomatoes cut into wedges (optional)
2oz (55g) alfalfa sprouts
1 tablespoon sunflower seeds
low-fat dressing of your choice (see pp. 53–4)

Combine all the ingredients for the salad and toss with the dressing of your choice just before serving.

Spinach and Tangerine Salad

serves 4–6

¹/₂lb (225g) fresh spinach, stems removed, washed and dried
4 mushrooms, cleaned, trimmed and sliced
2–3 tangerines, peeled and sectioned
2oz (55g) alfalfa sprouts or beansprouts (optional)
1 tablespoon chopped fresh tarragon, if available
1 recipe Low-fat Yoghurt Dressing (see p. 53)

Toss together the spinach, mushrooms, tangerine and alfalfa or beansprouts with the dressing and serve.

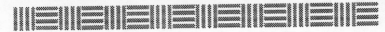

Marinated Vegetables

serves 6

Every few days make a bowl of these marinated vegetables to have on hand in the refrigerator for easy, delicious, healthy snacks, salads and sandwiches.

8oz (225g) mushrooms, cut in halves or quarters if large
1 cucumber, peeled and sliced
1 medium-sized courgette, sliced
1 cauliflower, broken into florets and steamed for 5 minutes
1 bunch broccoli, broken into florets and steamed for 5 minutes
1 sweet green pepper, sliced in rings
1 sweet red pepper, sliced in rings
1 red onion, sliced in rings

For the marinade
4fl. oz (120ml) wine or cider vinegar
juice of 1 large lemon
1–2 cloves garlic (to taste), finely chopped or put through a press
1 tablespoon Dijon mustard
1/2 teaspoon dried tarragon
1/2 teaspoon dried thyme or marjoram
2 tablespoons chopped fresh herbs, such as dill, basil, parsley or oregano
freshly ground pepper, to taste
3 tablespoons olive oil
1/2 pint (285ml) water

Prepare the vegetables and place them in a bowl.

Stir together the vinegar, lemon juice, garlic, mustard and herbs. Add freshly ground pepper to taste. Whisk in the olive oil and the water and combine thoroughly. Pour over the vegetables and toss together. Cover and refrigerate. This will keep for several days.

To serve as a salad, line plates with washed and dried lettuce leaves and top with the marinated vegetables. This also makes a delicious sandwich filling: see p. 49.

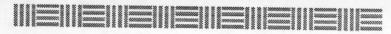

Broccoli Salad

serves 4

With the addition of tofu, this could be eaten as a main dish.

1 large bunch broccoli (1 1/2–2lb/680–900g), broken into florets, stems peeled and chopped
1 sweet red pepper, sliced
2 tablespoons freshly grated Parmesan or Gruyère cheese
2–4 tablespoons chopped fresh parsley or other herbs
4oz (115g) tofu, diced and tossed with soy sauce (optional)
low-fat dressing of your choice (see pp. 53–4)

Steam the broccoli for 5–8 minutes. Refresh under cold water and shake dry.

Toss with the remaining salad ingredients and the dressing of your choice. Serve, or chill and serve.

Batavia and Orange Salad

serves 4–6

In this, the sweet oranges contrast nicely with the bitter batavia lettuce.

1 small or 1/2 large batavia lettuce, leaves separated, washed well and dried
3 spring onions, sliced
4 radishes, cleaned and thinly sliced
4 mushrooms, cleaned, trimmed and sliced
2 oranges, rind and pith removed, cut into sections
1 recipe Low-fat Yoghurt Dressing (see p. 53)

Toss together the lettuce, spring onions, radishes, mushrooms and oranges with the dressing and serve.

Note You may add the juice of 1/2 orange to the dressing for a more orangey flavour.

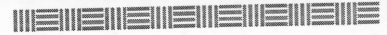

Tofu Salad

serves 4

12oz (340g) diced tofu
2–3 teaspoons soy sauce, to taste
1 teaspoon freshly grated ginger
1 green pepper, chopped
1 small onion, chopped
1 carrot, grated (optional)
3oz (85g) cucumber or celery, finely chopped
8fl. oz (225ml) either Low-fat Yoghurt Dressing or
    Curried Low-fat Dressing (see p. 53)

Wrap the tofu in a clean tea-towel and set it in a colander. Place a small cutting board over the tofu, and a pan of water on top of this to weight it down. Leave it for 30–60 minutes. The tofu will now be quite firm.

Toss together the tofu, soy sauce, ginger, chopped vegetables and dressing of your choice. Serve at once, or chill and serve. It will keep for about 3 days in the refrigerator.

This makes a good filling for sandwiches too: see p. 50.

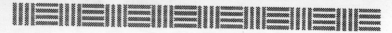

Tofu and Beansprout Salad

serves 4

4 oz (115g) tofu
soy sauce, to taste
4oz (115g) beansprouts
1 small green pepper, chopped
3 spring onions, chopped
1 tomato, chopped
1 tablespoon sesame or sunflower seeds (optional)
2–3 tablespoons chopped fresh coriander or other fresh herbs
1/2–1 teaspoon grated fresh ginger (optional)
6fl. oz (180ml) Low-fat Yoghurt Dressing, or Curried Low-fat Dressing or
  Tofu Dressing (see pp. 53–4)

Place the tofu in a bowl and mash it with the soy sauce. Toss with the remaining ingredients. Refrigerate in a covered bowl. Use for sandwiches, on wholemeal bread or pitta bread, or as a salad.

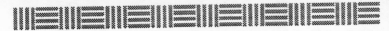

Oriental Beansprout Salad

serves 4–6

2oz (55g) alfalfa sprouts
4oz (115g) mung-bean sprouts or mixed beansprouts
2 tablespoons sunflower seeds
2 carrots, grated
2–3 spring onions, freshly chopped
2 tablespoons chopped fresh coriander

For the dressing

1 tablespoon sesame tahini
1 tablespoon soy sauce
4 tablespoons cider vinegar
1 teaspoon grated fresh ginger
1 clove garlic, finely chopped or put through a press
1 teaspoon Dijon mustard
freshly ground pepper, to taste
1 tablespoon sesame oil
3fl. oz (90ml) natural low-fat yoghurt or vegetable stock (see p. 80)

Toss together the ingredients for the salad.

Mix together the sesame tahini, soy sauce, vinegar, ginger, garlic, mustard and pepper. Whisk in the oil and the yoghurt or vegetable stock (this can be done in a blender). Blend well and toss with the salad mixture. Serve at once or chill in a covered container.

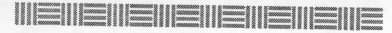

Middle Eastern Salad

serves 4–6

1 small cucumber, peeled and chopped
1 green pepper, chopped
4 medium-sized tomatoes, chopped
4 spring onions, chopped
1 tablespoon chopped fresh dill, if available
1 tablespoon chopped fresh parsley

For the dressing
juice of 1 large lemon
1–2 tablespoons red wine vinegar, to taste
1 small clove garlic, finely chopped or put through a press
1 teaspoon Dijon mustard (optional)
4fl. oz (120ml) natural low-fat yoghurt
freshly ground pepper, to taste

Toss together the vegetables and herbs.

Mix together the lemon juice, vinegar, garlic and mustard. Stir in the yoghurt and combine well. Add freshly ground pepper to taste. Serve at once, or chill and serve.

Warm Vegetable Salad

serves 6–8

1 red onion, cut in rings
1/2lb (225g) new potatoes, scrubbed and diced
1/2 bunch broccoli, cut into florets
1/2 head cauliflower, cut into florets
4oz (115g) mushrooms, cleaned, trimmed and quartered
12 cherry tomatoes
4oz (115g) cooked chick peas
1 recipe Low-fat Yoghurt Dressing (see p. 53)
4 tablespoons chopped fresh parsley or other herbs
2 tablespoons freshly grated Parmesan cheese

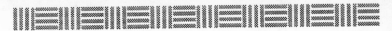

Place the onion and potatoes in a steamer above boiling water and steam for 10 minutes. Add the broccoli, cauliflower and mushrooms and continue to steam for 5–10 minutes, depending on how crunchy you want your vegetables. Remove from the heat, refresh under cold water and toss at once with the remaining ingredients. Serve warm.

This salad is excellent as a filling for sandwiches: see p. 50.

Grated Carrot Salad

serves 4–6

2lb (900g) carrots, peeled and grated
4–8 tablespoons chopped fresh parsley
1 recipe Low-fat Yoghurt Dressing or Curried Low-fat Dressing
  (see p. 53)

Toss together the carrots, parsley and dressing. Serve right away or refrigerate. This will keep for a couple of days in the refrigerator (you should add fresh parsley when you serve it, however).

Middle Eastern Version

Substitute the juice of 1 large orange for the dressing, and use 2 tablespoons chopped fresh mint instead of parsley.

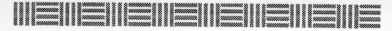

Carrot–Apple Salad

serves 4–6

1lb (450g) carrots, scrubbed and grated
1lb (450g) apples, grated
2 tablespoons currants

For the dressing
juice of ½ lemon
2 tablespoons cider vinegar
1 tablespoon apple juice
a pinch of salt
4fl. oz (120ml) natural low-fat yoghurt

Toss together the carrots, apples and currants.

Blend together the lemon juice, vinegar, apple juice and salt. Stir in the yoghurt. Toss with the carrots, apples and currants and serve.

Tomato Salad

serves 4–6

4 large, firm, ripe tomatoes, sliced thin
2 tablespoons chopped fresh herbs, such as basil, parsley, thyme, marjoram or dill
1 small clove garlic, finely chopped or put through a press
salt and freshly ground pepper, to taste
1–2 tablespoons balsamic vinegar, to taste
1 tablespoon olive oil (optional)

Slice the tomatoes and line a serving plate with them. Sprinkle with the herbs, garlic and salt and freshly ground pepper to taste. Drizzle on the vinegar and oil and serve.

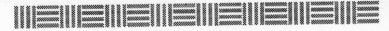

Watercress and Mushroom Salad

serves 4–6

2 large bunches watercress, washed, dried, stems trimmed
6oz (170g) mushrooms, trimmed, cleaned and sliced thin
1 recipe Low-fat Yoghurt Dressing or Tofu Dressing (see pp. 53–4)
handful alfalfa sprouts (about ½oz/15g)

Toss together the watercress and mushrooms with the dressing just before serving. Garnish with the alfalfa sprouts.

Warm Potato Salad

serves 6

1½lb (680g) new or russet potatoes, scrubbed
4 tablespoons dry white wine
1 red onion, thinly sliced
2 teaspoons caraway seeds
4 tablespoons chopped fresh parsley
2 tablespoons freshly grated Parmesan cheese (optional)
salt and freshly ground pepper, to taste
1 recipe Low-fat Yoghurt Dressing (see p. 53)

Cut the potatoes in half if large and steam until just tender: about 20 minutes. Refresh under cold water, dice and toss with the white wine. Add the onion, caraway seeds, parsley and optional Parmesan. Add salt and freshly ground pepper to taste.
   Mix together the dressing, toss with the salad and serve.

Note You can vary the flavour of this salad by adding 1 teaspoon curry powder or 1 teaspoon ground cumin to the vinaigrette.

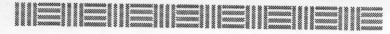

Mexican Rice Salad

serves 6–8

1/2lb (225g) white or brown rice
3/4 pint (425ml) water
1/2 teaspoon saffron threads, or 1/4 teaspoon saffron powder
salt and freshly ground pepper, to taste
1/2 lb (225g) green beans, trimmed and blanched
1 red pepper, seeded and cut into thin strips
4 spring onions, chopped
1 small cucumber, peeled, seeded and chopped
4 tablespoons chopped fresh coriander, to taste
1 hot green chilli, finely chopped (optional)

For the dressing
3 tablespoons wine or cider vinegar
juice of 1 large lemon
1 clove garlic, finely chopped or put through a press
1 teaspoon Dijon mustard
1 teaspoon ground cumin
4fl. oz (120ml) natural low-fat yoghurt
2fl. oz (60ml) olive oil
salt and freshly ground pepper, to taste
lettuce leaves, for the serving bowl or platter (optional)

Cook the rice in the water with the saffron and salt to taste. Meanwhile prepare the vegetables and the dressing.

For the dressing, mix together the vinegar, lemon juice, garlic, mustard and ground cumin. Blend in the yoghurt and oil, and combine well. Add salt and freshly ground pepper to taste.

Allow the rice to cool, then toss with the vegetables, coriander and the dressing. Chill for an hour or two, adjust the seasonings and serve, lining the bowl or serving platter, if you wish, with lettuce leaves.

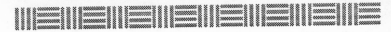

Mexican Corn Salad

serves 4

12oz (340g) cooked corn kernels (from 4 ears of corn, or use frozen)
1 green pepper, chopped
1 hot green chilli pepper, chopped
1 small onion, chopped
1/2 sweet red pepper, chopped
2 medium-sized ripe tomatoes, chopped
3 tablespoons chopped fresh coriander
2 oz (55g) cubed or grated skimmed-milk Mozzarella or any dry
    crumbly white cheese
1 recipe Low-fat Yoghurt Dressing (see p. 53) with 1/2–1 teaspoon
    ground cumin added
freshly ground pepper, to taste

Toss together all the vegetables, the fresh coriander and the cheese with
the dressing and serve, or chill and serve.

Curried Brown Rice Salad

serves 4

1/2lb (225g) brown rice, cooked
4oz (115g) mangetouts, steamed until bright green and crisp–tender
3 spring onions, chopped
1 stick celery, chopped
3oz (85g) cucumber, chopped
1 small green pepper, chopped
2 tablespoons grated Parmesan cheese
2 tablespoons sunflower seeds
8fl. oz (225ml) Curried Low-fat Dressing (see p. 53)

Cook the brown rice and toss it with the remaining ingredients.
Refrigerate for at least 1 hour in a covered container. This makes a good
lunch and will keep for 3 days in the refrigerator.

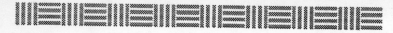

Lentil Salad

serves 4

¹/₂lb (225g) lentils, washed and picked over
1 small onion, chopped
2 cloves garlic, finely chopped
1 bay leaf
1¹/₄ pints (750ml) water
salt, to taste
6fl. oz (180ml) Low-fat Yoghurt Dressing (see p. 53)
¹/₂–1 teaspoon ground cumin (optional)
1 small green pepper, chopped
3 spring onions, chopped
3–4 tablespoons chopped fresh herbs, such as parsley, thyme,
    basil or coriander
freshly ground pepper, to taste

Combine the lentils, onion, garlic, bay leaf and water and bring to a boil.
Cover, reduce the heat and simmer for 45 minutes, until tender. Add salt
to taste. Drain off excess liquid (save it for soups) and remove the bay
leaf.

Make the dressing and stir in the optional cumin. Toss with the lentils,
green pepper, spring onions, and herbs. Add plenty of freshly ground
pepper.

Serve warm, or chill for several hours in a covered container. This will
keep for 5 days in the refrigerator.

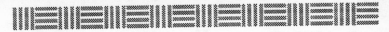

Millet–Lentil Salad

serves 4–6

6oz (170g) millet, cooked
5oz (140g) lentils, washed and cooked
2–3 medium-sized tomatoes, diced
4–6 spring onions, thinly sliced
1oz (30g) chopped fresh parsley
lettuce leaves, for garnish

For the dressing
4fl. oz (120ml) lemon juice
1 clove garlic, finely chopped or put through a press
1 teaspoon curry powder (or more, to taste)
1/2 teaspoon ground cumin
1/4 teaspoon ground coriander
1 teaspoon grated fresh ginger (optional)
salt and freshly ground pepper, to taste
8fl. oz (225ml) natural low-fat yoghurt

Mix together all the ingredients for the dressing and blend well.

Toss together the millet, lentils, tomatoes, spring onions and parsley.
Toss with the dressing, cover and chill for an hour or two. Serve on a bed
of lettuce leaves.

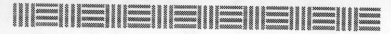

Bulgur Pilaf Salad

serves 4–6

4–8oz (115–225g) tofu, to taste
soy sauce, to taste
2 heaped cupfuls Bulgur Pilaf (see p. 169)
¾lb (340g) broccoli, steamed and chopped
2 tomatoes, chopped
4 tablespoons chopped fresh parsley (or more, to taste)

For the dressing
juice of 2 lemons
1 clove garlic, finely chopped or put through a press
1 teaspoon Dijon mustard
4fl. oz (120ml) plain low-fat yoghurt
freshly ground pepper, to taste

Mash the tofu with the soy sauce and toss with the Bulgur Pilaf, broccoli, tomatoes and parsley.

Mix together the lemon juice, garlic, mustard, yoghurt and freshly ground pepper and toss with the bulgur mixture. Refrigerate until ready to eat. This will keep for a couple of days in the refrigerator.

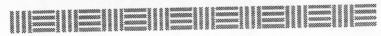

Tabouli

serves 6

I have used yoghurt in the dressing of this tabouli to add extra protein, so this would be viable as a main course.

½lb (225g) medium-grain bulgur wheat
boiling water to cover
1 small cucumber, chopped
4 spring onions, chopped
2oz (30g) chopped fresh parsley
4–6 tablespoons chopped fresh mint, to taste
4 tomatoes, chopped

For the dressing
juice of 2 large lemons (or more, to taste)
1 clove garlic, finely chopped or put through a press
1 teaspoon Dijon mustard (optional)
½ teaspoon ground cumin (optional)
salt and freshly ground pepper, to taste
2 tablespoons olive oil
4fl. oz (120ml) natural low-fat yoghurt

Place the bulgur in a bowl and pour on boiling water to cover by about 1 inch. Prepare the vegetables and dressing while the bulgur 'cooks' in the water.

For the dressing, mix together the lemon juice, garlic, mustard, cumin, salt and freshly ground pepper. Whisk in the olive oil and the yoghurt.

When the bulgur is soft pour off any excess water and press the bulgur in a strainer or squeeze it in a tea-towel. Then toss it with the cucumber, onions, parsley, mint, tomatoes and the dressing. Taste and adjust the seasonings, adding more lemon juice, garlic, mustard or salt and pepper if you wish. Refrigerate for several hours, or serve at once. This will keep for several days in the refrigerator.

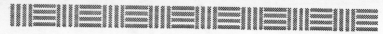

Warm Chick-pea Salad

serves 6

1lb (450g) chick peas, washed and picked over, or 3 tins (see note below)
2½ pints (1.5 litres) water (if using dried beans)
salt, to taste
4 spring onions, chopped
4 radishes, chopped
1 green or sweet red pepper, chopped
8 tablespoons chopped fresh parsley
1oz (30g) freshly grated Parmesan or Cheddar cheese
1 recipe Low-fat Yoghurt Dressing, plain or with cumin or curry, to
    taste (see p. 53)
freshly ground pepper, to taste
lettuce leaves, washed and dried, for serving

Pick over the chick peas, wash and soak for several hours or overnight in
the water. Drain them and place in a large pan with another 2½ pints (1.5
litres) water. Bring to the boil, cover and reduce the heat. Cook for 1–2
hours, until the chick peas are soft, adding salt to taste halfway through
the cooking.

Drain the chick peas and toss with the spring onions, radishes, green or
red pepper, parsley and grated cheese. Toss again with the dressing of
your choice and season to taste with freshly ground pepper. Serve warm,
on plates or from a bowl lined with lettuce leaves.

Note You can use tinned chick peas for this recipe. Simply heat the beans
in their liquid, drain and toss with the remaining ingredients.

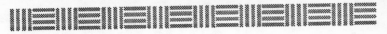

Mixed Bean Salad

serves 6–8

You can use tinned beans for this salad, or cook them yourself. If using tinned beans, retain the liquid for the dressing.

½lb (225g) each cooked chick peas, red kidney beans, and haricot or
  black beans
1 large sweet green pepper, chopped
1 small onion, chopped, or 4 spring onions, chopped
1–2 hot green chilli peppers, finely chopped
3–4 tablespoons chopped coriander

For the dressing
4 tablespoons wine or cider vinegar
1 clove garlic, finely chopped or put through a press
1 teaspoon Dijon mustard
½–1 teaspoon ground cumin, to taste
6fl. oz (180ml) liquid from the beans
salt and freshly ground pepper, to taste

Mix together the beans, green pepper, onion, chilli peppers and coriander.
  For the dressing, mix together the vinegar, garlic, mustard and cumin. Stir in the liquid from the beans and combine well. Add salt and freshly ground pepper to taste.
  Toss the dressing with the beans and serve, or chill and serve.

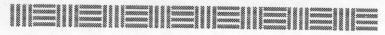

Low-fat Egg Salad

serves 4

4 hard-boiled eggs, chopped
whites only of 4 additional hard-boiled eggs, chopped
1 green pepper, finely chopped
1 small onion, finely chopped
1 stick celery, finely chopped
3 tablespoons chopped fresh parsley
1 recipe Low-fat Yoghurt Dressing or Tofu Dressing (see pp. 53–4)
1–3 teaspoons additional Dijon mustard
freshly ground pepper, to taste
1/2 teaspoon paprika or curry powder (optional)

Toss together the chopped eggs and egg whites with the vegetables,
parsley, dressing, additional mustard, ground pepper and optional paprika
or curry powder. Store in the refrigerator in a covered container, and use
for sandwiches or salads.

Chicken Salad

serves 4

12oz (340g) cooked chicken breast, diced
1 green pepper, chopped
1 small onion, chopped
3oz (85g) cucumber or celery, chopped
8fl. oz (225ml) Low-fat Yoghurt Dressing or Curried Low-fat
   Dressing (see p. 53)
1 teaspoon freshly grated ginger (optional)
1/2–1 teaspoon soy sauce (optional)

Toss together the chicken, chopped vegetables and dressing of your
choice. Add fresh ginger and soy sauce as desired. Serve at once, or chill
and serve. This is good for sandwiches too. Try filling pitta breads with it.

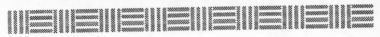

Chinese Chicken Salad

serves 4

12oz (340g) cooked chicken breast, diced
1 green pepper, chopped
4 spring onions, chopped
2 tablespoons sunflower or sesame seeds
3oz (85g) cucumber, chopped
3 tablespoons chopped fresh coriander

For the dressing
4 tablespoons white wine or cider vinegar, or lemon juice
1 tablespoon soy sauce
1 clove garlic, finely chopped or put through a press
2 teaspoons grated fresh ginger, or ½ teaspoon dried ginger
freshly ground pepper, to taste
2 tablespoons sesame oil
4fl. oz (120ml) natural low-fat yoghurt

Toss together the chicken, green pepper, spring onions, sunflower or sesame seeds, cucumber and fresh coriander.

Mix together the vinegar or lemon juice, the soy sauce, garlic and ginger. Add freshly ground pepper to taste. Whisk in the sesame oil and the yoghurt. Toss with the salad and serve, or refrigerate and serve. This will keep for a day or two in the refrigerator.

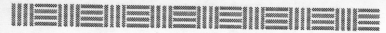

Cottage Cheese and Fruit Salad

serves 4

This makes a perfect lunch, light summer meal or substantial breakfast.

1lb (450g) low-fat cottage cheese
1 apple, chopped
1 banana or pear, chopped
4oz (115g) fresh pineapple, chopped
2 tablespoons sunflower seeds (optional)
2 tablespoons raisins
fresh mint, for garnish

Toss together all the ingredients and chill until ready to serve. Serve garnished with fresh mint.

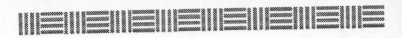

Soups

Soups make great diet meals. A substantial bowl of any of the soups here will be low in calories, yet quite filling and comforting.

Some of the soups here are hearty meals in themselves – soups like the Minestrone on p. 82, the Bean and Vegetable Soup on p. 85, or the Haricot Bean Soup on p. 84. Others make lighter meals or first courses. Accompany them with wholemeal bread and a salad, and you will be very satisfied indeed.

There is no need to thicken soups with cream, as is so often done in restaurants. The puréed vegetable soups in this section are thickened with potato, and the bean soups are partially or thoroughly puréed in a blender to make a rich, creamy potage.

If you wish, you can double or even triple soup recipes and eat them throughout the week. You could begin a big vegetable soup on a Sunday, say, and add different vegetables and/or beans, grains and/or pasta to it throughout the week. These soups also freeze well, if you wish to double quantities for the freezer.

Garlic Broth

2¹/₂–3 pints (1.5–2 litres)

This is an aromatic vegetable broth made by simmering garlic slowly in water. The pungency of the garlic is mollified by the slow cooking.

2 heads garlic, cloves separated and peeled
3 pints (2 litres) water
2–3 teaspoons salt, to taste
1 bay leaf
a pinch of dried thyme

Combine all the ingredients in a soup pot and bring to a simmer. Cover and simmer for 1–2 hours. Remove from the heat and strain. Discard the garlic, or purée it and use it as a spread on toast. Adjust the seasoning. Use the broth as a base for soups such as Minestrone (see p. 82) or vegetable soups. This freezes well.

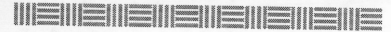

Vegetable Stock

3 pints (2 litres)

This is a mild, fragrant stock. The vegetables can be prepared quickly, and the stock requires no skimming. It freezes well.

3 pints (2 litres) plus 8fl. oz (225ml) water
2 large onions, peeled and quartered
6 large cloves garlic, peeled
2 large carrots, peeled and coarsely sliced
2 large potatoes, scrubbed and quartered
2 leeks, white parts only, cleaned and sliced thick
2 sticks celery, sliced thick
a *bouquet garni* made with 1 bay leaf, a couple of sprigs of fresh
    parsley and a few sprigs of fresh thyme
12 whole black peppercorns
about 1 teaspoon salt (or more, to taste)

Combine all the ingredients in a large soup pot and bring to the boil. Reduce the heat, cover and simmer for 1 hour. Strain and discard the vegetables.

Note   For a 'meatier'-tasting stock, add 1 tablespoon soy sauce and a couple of dried mushrooms, soaked for 30 minutes in warm water and rinsed thoroughly. Strain the mushroom-soaking liquid through a strainer lined with kitchen paper and add this to the stock.

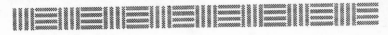

Low-fat Chicken Stock

2¹/₂ pints (1.5 litres)

carcass and giblets of 1 chicken, very fresh, plus 2–4 extra wings; or the
   carcass of a cooked chicken
1 carrot, sliced
1 onion, quartered
5 cloves garlic, peeled and crushed
a *bouquet garni* made with 1 bay leaf, a couple of sprigs of fresh
  thyme, and a couple of sprigs of fresh parsley
1 stick celery, sliced
3 pints (2 litres) plus 8fl. oz (225ml) water
¹/₂ teaspoon black peppercorns
salt, to taste

Crack the chicken bones slightly with a hammer if using an uncooked
carcass, and combine them with the remaining ingredients in a soup pot.
  Bring to the boil and skim off any scum that rises. Reduce the heat,
cover the pot and simmer for 1–2 hours. Strain, and discard the bones
and vegetables. Place the stock in a covered bowl in the refrigerator and
chill overnight. The next day, remove the stock from the refrigerator and
skim off any fat that has risen to the surface and congealed.

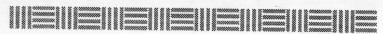

Minestrone

serves 6–8

This hearty *potage* can be a week-long soup. Every day add more vegetables and water, and you will keep it going. If you add different kinds of
vegetables each day you won't get tired of it.

1 tablespoon olive oil
1 onion, chopped
3–4 cloves garlic, finely chopped or put through a press
2 carrots, sliced
1/2 small green cabbage, shredded
3/4lb (340g) potatoes, scrubbed and diced
1lb (450g) tinned or fresh tomatoes, peeled and sliced
4 tablespoons tomato purée
3 pints (2 litres) vegetable stock (see p. 80) or water
1 rind from Parmesan cheese, if available (optional)
1 bay leaf
1 teaspoon dried oregano
1/2 teaspoon dried thyme
salt and freshly ground pepper, to taste
1 teaspoon dried basil, or 1 tablespoon fresh basil
1/2lb (225g) cooked haricot beans or chick peas
2 medium-sized courgettes, sliced
6oz (170g) peas, fresh or frozen
4oz (115g) broken spaghetti or flat noodles
3oz (85g) freshly grated Parmesan or Gruyère cheese
4 tablespoons chopped fresh parsley
3 tablespoons chopped fresh basil, if available

Heat the oil in a large, heavy-bottomed soup pot or casserole and add the
onion and garlic. Sauté until the onion is tender, then add the carrots and
cabbage. Sauté for about 1 minute and add the potatoes, tomatoes,
tomato purée and vegetable stock or water. Bring to a simmer and add
the optional rind of Parmesan (this gives the soup a great cheesy flavour
without additional cheese), the bay leaf, oregano, thyme, salt, basil and
cooked beans or chick peas. Simmer, covered, for 1 hour. Taste and adjust
seasonings, adding more garlic, salt or herbs if you wish. Season with lots
of freshly ground pepper.

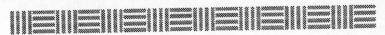

Add the courgettes and peas and simmer for 10–15 minutes. Add the spaghetti and continue to simmer until the pasta is cooked *al dente* – firm to the bite. Remove the Parmesan rind. Serve, topping each bowl with Parmesan or Gruyère and chopped fresh parsley and basil, if available.

Beetroot and Vegetable Borscht

serves 6

1 tablespoon safflower or sunflower oil
2 medium-sized onions, chopped
3 cloves garlic, finely chopped or put through a press
1lb (450g) raw beetroots, peeled and chopped
½lb (225g) green cabbage, shredded
2 sticks celery, sliced
1 carrot, peeled and finely chopped
½lb (225g) potatoes, scrubbed and diced
1 medium-sized sweet green or red pepper, chopped
½lb (225g) tomatoes, peeled and chopped
½ teaspoon dried thyme
½ teaspoon crushed dill seeds
salt and freshly ground pepper, to taste
3 pints (2 litres) vegetable stock (see p. 80) or water
juice of 1 large lemon
2–3 tablespoons chopped fresh dill, to taste
8fl. oz (225ml) natural low-fat yoghurt

Heat the oil in a large, heavy-bottomed soup pot and add the onion and garlic. Sauté for a few minutes, until the onion begins to soften, then add the beetroots, cabbage, celery, carrot, potatoes and red or green peppers. Sauté, stirring for a few minutes, then add the tomatoes, thyme, dill seeds, salt and freshly ground pepper to taste, and the water or stock. Bring to the boil, cover, reduce the heat and simmer for 1 hour.

Remove ½ pint (285ml) of the soup from the pot and purée it in a blender or food processor. Return it to the soup pot, stir in the dill and lemon juice. Correct the seasonings. Heat the soup through and serve, topping each bowl with a generous dollop of yoghurt.

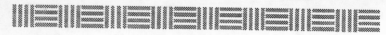

Haricot Bean Soup with Wholemeal Croûtons

serves 6

1 tablespoon safflower or olive oil
1 onion, chopped
3 cloves garlic, finely chopped or put through a press
1lb (450g) haricot beans, washed, picked over and soaked overnight
2½ pints (1.5 litres) water
1 bay leaf
½ teaspoon dried thyme
1–2 teaspoons salt, to taste
freshly ground pepper, to taste
up to 8fl. oz (225ml) skimmed milk (optional)
juice of 1 large lemon
4 tablespoons chopped fresh parsley
6 wholemeal garlic croûtons (see p. 92)

Heat the oil in a large, heavy-bottomed soup pot or casserole and sauté the onion and 2 cloves of the garlic until the onion is tender.

Drain the soaked beans and add to the pot, along with the water and bay leaf. Bring to the boil, reduce the heat and simmer for 1½ hours. Add the thyme, salt to taste and the remaining garlic and continue to simmer for another 30–60 minutes, until the beans are thoroughly tender. Remove the bay leaf and purée the soup in a blender. Return to the pot and heat through. Add freshly ground pepper to taste and adjust the salt. If you wish, thin out to the desired consistency with skimmed milk.

Just before serving, stir in the lemon juice. Serve, topping each bowl with parsley and croûtons.

Haricot Bean Soup Using Tinned Beans

For the beans and water substitute three 14oz (385g) tins haricot beans and 1¼ pints (750ml) water. Proceed as in the recipe above, sautéeing the onion and garlic in the oil, and adding the beans and their liquid. But you needn't bring this to a simmer. Purée and return to the pot, then proceed as above.

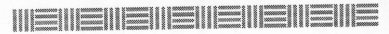

Bean and Vegetable Soup

serves 6

½lb (225g) dried borlotti beans, kidney beans or haricot beans,
   picked over, washed and soaked overnight or for several hours
1½ pints (850ml) water
1 bay leaf
1 tablespoon olive oil
2 medium-sized yellow onions, chopped
4 large cloves garlic, finely chopped or put through a press
2 sticks celery, diced
3 medium-sized carrots, peeled and diced
4 medium-sized potatoes, diced
1lb (450g) ripe tomatoes, chopped
1 tablespoon tomato purée
3lb (1.5kg) Swiss chard, stems removed, leaves cleaned and chopped
1lb (450g) spinach, kale or other greens, stems removed, leaves
   cleaned and chopped
1 hot dried red chilli pepper
1 teaspoon dried thyme
2–2½ pints (1.2–1.5 litres) additional water
the cooking water from the beans
salt and freshly ground pepper, to taste

Soak the beans overnight, drain and combine them with 1½ pints (850ml) water in a soup pot or large saucepan. Bring to the boil, add the bay leaf, reduce the heat, cover and simmer for 1–2 hours, until tender. Add salt to taste to the cooking liquid, drain the beans and retain the liquid. Purée half the beans in some of their cooking liquid in a blender or food processor fitted with the steel blade, and set aside.

Heat the olive oil in a large, heavy-bottomed soup pot over a low heat and add the onion and half the garlic. Sauté, stirring, for about 5 minutes, then add the celery and carrots. Sauté, stirring, for another 10 minutes, and add all the remaining vegetables, the tomato purée, hot chilli pepper, the whole cooked beans, the thyme, the remaining water and the cooking liquid from the beans. Add some salt, bring to a simmer, cover and simmer for 1 hour. If the vegetables aren't covered, add another cup of water. Stir in the puréed beans and the remaining garlic, and mix well. Add salt and freshly ground pepper to taste, and more thyme or garlic if you wish. Heat through and serve.

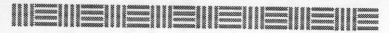

Split-pea Soup

serves 6

1 tablespoon sunflower, safflower or olive oil
1 medium-sized onion, chopped
2 cloves garlic, finely chopped or put through a press
2 sticks celery, chopped
1 carrot, chopped
1lb (450g) split peas, washed and picked over
3 pints (2 litres) water
1 bay leaf
1/2 teaspoon dried thyme
salt and freshly ground pepper, to taste
4fl. oz (120ml) natural low-fat yoghurt

Heat the oil in a heavy-bottomed soup pot and sauté the onion and one clove of the garlic until the onion is tender. Add the carrot and celery, sauté for another minute and add the split peas, water and bay leaf. Bring to the boil, reduce the heat and simmer for 1 hour. Add the remaining garlic, the thyme and salt to taste, and simmer for another 30 minutes. Purée half the soup in a blender and return it to the pot. Heat it through, adjust the seasonings, adding more salt or garlic if you wish and lots of freshly ground pepper. Serve piping hot, topping each bowl with a spoonful of yoghurt.

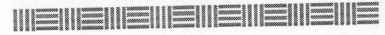

Indian Split-pea Soup

serves 4

1 tablespoon black peppercorns
12 cloves
1 bay leaf, crushed
1 tablespoon safflower or sunflower oil
1 small onion, finely chopped
1 teaspoon mustard seeds
1/2lb (225g) green or yellow split peas, washed and picked over
1/2 teaspoon turmeric
2 pints (1.2 litres) vegetable stock (see p. 80) or water
salt and freshly ground pepper, to taste
2 tablespoons milk (optional)
juice of 1/2 lemon
1 lemon, cut into wedges, for garnish
natural low-fat yoghurt, for garnish (optional)
4 tablespoons garlic croûtons (see p. 92) for garnish

Tie the black peppercorns, the cloves and the bay leaf in a cheesecloth and set aside.

Heat the oil in a heavy-bottomed soup pot or casserole and sauté the onion with the mustard seeds over a medium heat until the onion is tender. Add the split peas, the turmeric, the stock or water, salt to taste and the spices in their cheesecloth bag. Bring to a boil, reduce the heat and simmer for 45–60 minutes, until the peas are tender.

Remove the cheesecloth bag from the soup and squeeze out all the liquid. Purée the soup in a blender or put it through a food mill. Return it to the pot and heat through.

Correct the seasonings, adding salt and freshly ground pepper to taste, and stir in the optional milk. Serve, sprinkling fresh lemon juice over each bowl and garnishing with lemon wedges, croûtons and the optional natural low-fat yoghurt.

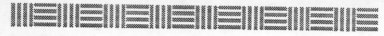

Hearty Lentil Soup

serves 4–6

1 tablespoon safflower, sunflower or olive oil
1 onion, chopped
4 cloves garlic, finely chopped or put through a press
1lb (450g) lentils, washed and picked over
2 carrots, chopped
2 medium-sized potatoes, chopped
2 medium-sized tomatoes, chopped
3 pints (2 litres) water
1 bay leaf
1 teaspoon cumin
a pinch of cayenne
1/2 teaspoon dried oregano or thyme
salt and freshly ground pepper, to taste
more water, as needed
chopped fresh parsley, for garnish

Heat the oil in a heavy-bottomed soup pot and add the onion and 2 cloves of the garlic. Sauté until the onion is tender and add the lentils, carrots, potatoes, tomatoes, water, bay leaf and cumin. Bring to the boil, reduce the heat, cover and simmer for 30 minutes. Add the remaining garlic, the cayenne, oregano or thyme, salt to taste and lots of freshly ground pepper, then simmer for another 15–30 minutes. Remove 3/4 pint (425ml) of the soup and purée it in a blender. Stir it back into the soup. Heat through, correct the seasonings and serve, garnishing each serving with chopped fresh parsley.

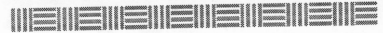

Puréed Lentil Soup

serves 6

1 tablespoon olive oil
1 large onion, chopped
4 cloves garlic, finely chopped or put through a press
1 stick celery, chopped
14oz (395g) green or brown lentils, washed and picked over
3 pints (2 litres) water
1 bay leaf
salt and freshly ground pepper, to taste
juice of ½–1 lemon (optional)
1–2 teaspoons ground cumin, to taste
2–3 tablespoons chopped fresh parsley

Heat the oil in a heavy-bottomed soup pot and sauté the onion and garlic until the onion begins to colour. Add the celery and sauté for another few minutes, then add the lentils, water and bay leaf. Bring to the boil, reduce the heat, cover and cook for 30–40 minutes, until the lentils are tender. Add salt and freshly ground pepper to taste, lemon juice if you wish, and the cumin, then simmer for another 5–10 minutes. Remove the bay leaf.

Remove the soup from the heat and purée all of it or some of it (depending on how thick you want it) in a blender or using the fine blade of a food mill. Return it to the pot and heat through, stirring. If the soup seems too watery, simmer a bit longer to reduce it, making sure to stir it often so that it doesn't stick to the bottom of the pot. Adjust seasonings and serve, garnished with parsley.

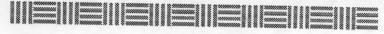

Chick-pea and Tomato Soup

serves 6

1lb (450g) chick peas, picked over, washed and soaked overnight
2½ pints (1.5 litres) water
1 tablespoon olive oil
1 large onion, chopped
3 large cloves garlic (or more, to taste), finely chopped or put
    through a press
1lb (450g) fresh or tinned tomatoes, chopped
2 tablespoons tomato purée
1 bay leaf
1 small dried hot red pepper, such as cayenne
½ teaspoon dried thyme
½–1 teaspoon dried oregano
½ teaspoon dried rosemary
salt and freshly ground pepper, to taste
chopped fresh parsley, for garnish

Combine the soaked chick peas with 2½ pints (1.5 litres) water, bring to
the boil, reduce the heat and simmer, covered, for 1 hour.

Heat the olive oil in a heavy-bottomed soup pot or casserole and sauté
the onion and 1 clove of the garlic until the onion is tender. Add the chick
peas with their cooking liquid, the remaining garlic, the tomatoes, tomato
purée, bay leaf and hot red pepper, thyme, oregano, rosemary and salt,
and bring to a boil. Reduce the heat, cover and simmer for 1–2 hours,
until the beans are tender. Add more water if the soup seems too thick.
Add pepper and adjust the seasonings. Serve garnished with chopped
fresh parsley.

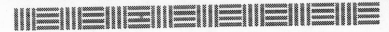

Hearty Mushroom and Barley Soup

serves 6

1 tablespoon olive oil
1 medium-sized onion, chopped
2 large cloves garlic, finely chopped or put through a press
8oz (225g) mushrooms, cleaned, trimmed and sliced
3 tablespoons dry white wine
1 tablespoon soy sauce
½ teaspoon dried thyme (or more, to taste)
½ teaspoon crumbled dried rosemary (or more, to taste)
¾lb (340g) barley, washed
3 pints (2 litres) vegetable stock (see p. 80) or *bouillon*
salt and freshly ground pepper, to taste
1–2 tablespoons dry sherry, to taste
2–3 tablespoons chopped fresh dill or parsley
4fl. oz (120ml) natural low-fat yoghurt, for garnish (optional)

Heat the oil in a heavy-bottomed soup pot and sauté the onion and
1 clove of the garlic until the onion begins to soften. Add the mushrooms
and remaining garlic and sauté, stirring over a medium heat for about 5
minutes, until the mushrooms release some of their liquid. Add the wine
and soy sauce, the thyme and rosemary, and sauté for another few minutes. Add the barley and sauté, stirring for about 3 minutes, until the grains
are coated with oil. Add the stock or broth and bring to the boil. Reduce
the heat, cover and simmer for 40 minutes, or until the barley is tender
and the soup fragrant. Add salt and pepper to taste, and a tablespoon
or two of dry sherry. Just before serving, stir in the chopped fresh dill or
parsley.

Serve, topping each serving with natural low-fat yoghurt if desired.

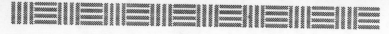

Provençal Garlic Soup

serves 4

2 pints (1.2 litres) water
6 large cloves garlic, finely chopped or put through a press
1–2 teaspoons salt, to taste
½ teaspoon dried thyme
4 leaves fresh sage, chopped, or ½ teaspoon dried sage (optional)
1 bay leaf
2 eggs
2 tablespoons chopped fresh parsley
4–6 garlic croûtons (see below)

Bring the water to a boil and add the garlic, salt, thyme, sage and bay leaf. Simmer for 10–15 minutes. Adjust the seasonings.

Beat the egg in a bowl and ladle in some hot soup. Stir together, then stir back into the soup. Serve at once, topping each bowl with parsley and a garlic croûton.

Garlic Croûtons

Toast pieces of wholemeal bread and rub at once with the cut side of a clove of garlic.

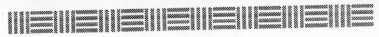

Curried Cauliflower Soup

serves 4–6

1 tablespoon safflower or sunflower oil
1 onion, chopped
1 clove garlic, finely chopped or put through a press
1–2 teaspoons curry powder, to taste
1/2–1 teaspoon ground cumin, to taste
1 small head cauliflower, broken into florets
2 pints (1.2 litres) vegetable stock, chicken stock (see pp. 80 and 81) or
   bouillon
1 small potato, peeled and diced
salt, to taste
freshly ground pepper, to taste
8fl. oz (225ml) natural low-fat yoghurt
1 teaspoon cornflour
chopped fresh coriander, for garnish
fresh lemon juice, to taste (optional)

Heat the oil in a soup pot and sauté the onion and garlic until the onion is tender. Add the curry powder, cumin and the cauliflower, stir together for a minute or two, then add the stock or *bouillon* and the potato and bring to the boil. Cover, reduce the heat and simmer for 30–45 minutes. Purée in a blender or food processor, in batches. Return to the pot and adjust the seasonings, adding salt, pepper and more curry powder or cumin to taste. Heat through.

Stir together the yoghurt and cornflour and whisk it into the soup. Heat through, but don't boil, and serve, garnishing with chopped fresh coriander and a sprinkle of lemon juice if you wish.

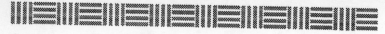

Potato–Leek Soup

serves 4–6

1 tablespoon olive oil
4 leeks, white part only, washed well and sliced
3 pints (2 litres) vegetable stock, chicken stock (see pp. 80 and 81) water
   or *bouillon*
2lb (900g) potatoes, scrubbed and diced
1/4 teaspoon dried thyme
salt and freshly ground pepper, to taste
2 tablespoons dry white wine
1oz (30g) grated Gruyère or Parmesan cheese (optional)
fresh chopped parsley, for garnish

Heat the oil in a heavy-bottomed soup pot and sauté the leeks over a low
heat, stirring from time to time, for 10–15 minutes. Add the water or
stock, potatoes and thyme, and bring to a simmer. Cover and simmer for
30–45 minutes. Add salt and freshly ground pepper to taste, and the wine.
Correct the seasonings and serve, topping each bowl with optional grated
cheese and chopped fresh parsley.

Puréed Potato and Parsley Soup

serves 4

1 1/2 pints (850ml) water
1lb (450g) potatoes, peeled and quartered
1 onion, peeled and quartered
4 whole cloves garlic, peeled but not crushed
salt and freshly ground pepper, to taste
1 large bunch parsley, washed, stems removed
1/2 pint (285ml) skimmed milk (or more, for a thinner soup)

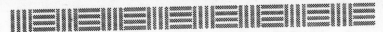

Combine the water, potatoes, onion, garlic and some salt in a saucepan or soup pot and bring to the boil. Cover, reduce the heat and simmer for 45 minutes, or until the potatoes and onion are quite tender. Remove from the heat and purée, along with the parsley, in a blender. Add the milk and return the soup to the pot. Heat through, stirring. Taste, add salt and freshly ground pepper to taste, and serve.

Corn Chowder

serves 6–8

This is an American classic, altered here to make a low-fat recipe.

1 tablespoon safflower or sunflower oil
1 onion, chopped
1 medium or large sweet green pepper, chopped
2 medium-sized potatoes, scrubbed and diced
1lb (225g) fresh or frozen corn kernels (from 4–5 ears corn)
1½ pints (850ml) water or vegetable stock (see p. 80)
½ teaspoon dried thyme
1 pint (570ml) skimmed milk
salt and freshly ground pepper, to taste
2oz (55g) grated Gruyère cheese
4 tablespoons chopped fresh parsley or coriander, for garnish

Heat the oil in a heavy-bottomed soup pot or casserole and sauté the onion and green pepper until the onion is tender. Add the potatoes, corn and water or vegetable stock and bring to the boil. Reduce the heat, cover and simmer for 45 minutes. Purée half the soup very coarsely in a blender or food processor. Return to the pot and add the thyme, milk, and salt and freshly ground pepper to taste. Heat through for about 10 minutes, then stir in the grated cheese. Correct the seasonings and serve, topping each bowl with chopped fresh parsley or coriander.

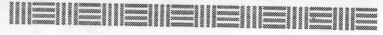

Purée of Spinach Soup

serves 4

1 tablespoon sunflower, safflower or olive oil
1 small onion, chopped
1 clove garlic, finely chopped or put through a press
1 lb (450g) fresh spinach, washed, stemmed and chopped; or
    a 10oz (285g) packet frozen spinach
1 large potato, peeled and diced
1¼ pint (750ml) water, vegetable stock or chicken stock (see pp. 80 and
    81)
salt and freshly ground pepper, to taste
¾ pint (425ml) skimmed milk
a pinch of nutmeg
2oz (55g) freshly grated Parmesan or Gruyère cheese
4fl. oz (120ml) natural low-fat yoghurt

Heat the oil in a large, heavy-bottomed soup pot or casserole and sauté
the onion and garlic until the onion is tender. Add the spinach, potato and
water or stock and bring to the boil. Add salt to taste, reduce the heat,
cover and simmer for 20 minutes, or until the potato is tender. Purée in
a blender or put through a food mill, then return to the pot. Add the milk
and nutmeg and heat through. Add freshly ground pepper to taste, adjust
the salt, stir in the grated cheese and serve, topping each bowl with a dollop of low-fat yoghurt.

Fresh Pea Soup

serves 4

¾ pint (425ml) water
1 medium-sized potato, peeled and diced
1¼lb (565g) peas, fresh or frozen
1 pint (570ml) skimmed milk
3 tablespoons dry white wine
salt and freshly ground pepper, to taste
1–2 tablespoons chopped fresh parsley or chervil
4fl. oz (120ml) natural low-fat yoghurt, for garnish

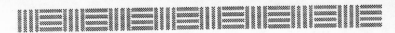

Combine the water and potato and salt to taste, and bring to the boil. Cover, reduce the heat and simmer for 20 minutes. Add the peas. Simmer for another 5–10 minutes, until the peas are tender but still bright green. Remove from the heat and purée in a blender or food processor, or put through a food mill. Return to the pot and stir in the milk and the dry white wine. Heat through, stirring. Correct the seasonings, adding freshly ground pepper to taste, and stir in the chopped fresh herbs. Serve, garnishing each bowl with natural low-fat yoghurt.

Courgette Soup with Dill

serves 4

2lb (900g) courgettes, sliced
1 tablespoon olive oil
1 small onion, chopped
1 clove garlic, finely chopped or put through a press
1 ½ pints (850ml) vegetable stock or chicken stock (see pp. 80 and 81)
2–3 tablespoons chopped fresh dill, to taste
lemon juice, to taste
salt and freshly ground pepper, to taste
4 tablespoons natural low-fat yoghurt, for garnish (optional)

Steam the courgettes for 10 minutes. Refresh under cold water.
    Meanwhile, heat the oil in a frying pan and sauté the garlic and onion until the onion is tender. Set aside.
    Purée the steamed courgettes, with the onion and garlic and some stock to moisten, in a blender or food processor. Transfer to a soup pot and stir in the remaining stock. Heat through over a medium heat and stir in the dill, lemon juice and salt and freshly ground pepper to taste.
    Serve, garnishing each bowl with a dollop of natural low-fat yoghurt.

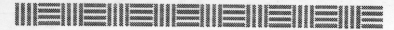

Puréed Pumpkin Soup

serves 4

1 tablespoon safflower or sunflower oil
1 small onion, chopped
1 medium-sized clove garlic, finely chopped or put through a press
2½lb (1.25kg) pumpkin, peeled and diced
1 medium-sized potato, peeled and diced
2½ pints (1.5 litres) water or vegetable stock (see p. 80)
salt and freshly ground pepper, to taste
1 teaspoon dried thyme
4 tablespoons natural low-fat yoghurt, for garnish

Heat the oil in a large, heavy-bottomed soup pot and sauté the onion and garlic until the onion starts to become tender. Add the pumpkin and potato and sauté for another 2–3 minutes. Add the water or stock and some salt, and bring to a simmer. Cover and simmer for 30 minutes.

Purée the soup through a food mill or in a blender or food processor. Return to the pot and add the thyme, pepper and more salt to taste. Heat through, adjust the seasonings and serve, garnishing each bowl with a dollop of yoghurt.

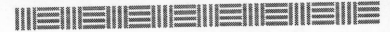

Tomato Soup with Coriander

serves 4

1 tablespoon olive oil
1 onion, chopped
2 cloves garlic, finely chopped or put through a press
1 1/2 teaspoons paprika
a 28oz (790g) tin tomatoes, chopped, with juice
1 1/2 pints (850ml) water
2 tablespoons tomato purée
2 whole bunches fresh coriander
salt and freshly ground pepper, to taste
1oz (30g) vermicelli
a pinch of cayenne
juice of 1 lime (or more, to taste)

Tie the bunches of coriander together so that you can remove them after
the soup simmers.

Heat the olive oil in a large, heavy-bottomed soup pot or casserole and
sauté the onion over a medium–low heat until tender.

Add the garlic and paprika, sauté for 1 minute, then add the tomatoes
and their juice, the water, the tomato purée, coriander, and salt and freshly
ground pepper to taste. Bring to a simmer, cover and simmer for 30 minutes.

Remove the soup from the heat. Take out the coriander bunches and
discard them, and put the soup in a blender or through a food mill. Return
it to the heat, bring it back to a simmer and add the vermicelli. Simmer
until the vermicelli is cooked *al dente* – firm to the bite – add the cayenne,
adjust the seasonings and stir in the lime juice. Serve at once.

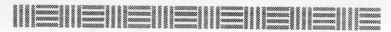

Curried Cabbage and Apple Soup

serves 4–6

1 tablespoon safflower or sunflower oil
1 large onion, chopped
2 cloves garlic, finely chopped or put through a press
1lb (450g) red or green cabbage, shredded
2½ pints (1.5 litres) water or vegetable stock (see p. 80)
1–2 teaspoons curry powder
1 tablespoon soy sauce (or more, to taste)
salt and freshly ground pepper, to taste
2 tart apples, cored and sliced
8fl. oz (225ml) natural low-fat yoghurt

For garnish

4–6 tablespoons additional yoghurt
½ additional apple, sliced thin and tossed with lemon juice

Heat the oil in a heavy-bottomed soup pot or casserole and sauté the
onion and garlic over a medium heat, until the onion begins to soften. Add
the cabbage and sauté for another 5 minutes, stirring. Add the water or
stock, the curry powder, soy sauce and salt to taste. Bring to the boil,
reduce the heat, cover and simmer for 30 minutes. Add the apples and
continue to simmer for another 15–20 minutes. Taste and adjust the seasoning, adding more salt or curry powder to taste. Remove from the heat,
cool for a minute, then stir in the yoghurt and freshly ground pepper to
taste. Serve, topping each bowl with a spoonful of yoghurt and a few slices
of apple.

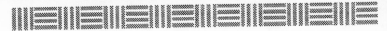

Red Cabbage and Apple Soup

serves 4–6

1 tablespoon safflower or sunflower oil
1 medium-sized onion, chopped
1 clove garlic, finely chopped or put through a press
1 teaspoon cinnamon
1/4 teaspoon ground cloves
1/2 teaspoon allspice
1lb (450g) red cabbage, shredded
2 1/2 pints (1.5 litres) water
salt, to taste
freshly ground pepper, to taste
2 tart apples, cored and sliced
8fl. oz (225ml) natural low-fat yoghurt, for garnish
1/2 additional apple, sliced thin and tossed with lemon juice, for garnish

Heat the oil in a heavy-bottomed soup pot and sauté the onion and garlic over a medium heat until the onion begins to soften. Add the spices and sauté for another 2–3 minutes, stirring. Add the cabbage and sauté for 5 minutes, stirring. Add the water and salt to taste, bring to the boil, reduce the heat, cover and simmer for 30 minutes.

Add the apples and continue to simmer for another 15–20 minutes. Taste and adjust the seasoning, adding more salt or spices to taste. Serve, stirring yoghurt into each serving and topping with a few slices of apple tossed with lemon juice.

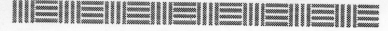

Cabbage Soup Chinoise

serves 4

This very light soup is made in minutes.

2 pints (1.2 litres) vegetable stock, chicken stock (see pp. 80 and 81)
   or *bouillon*
1lb (450g) Chinese cabbage, shredded
6 spring onions, thinly sliced
4 tablespoons soy sauce
2 tablespoons dry sherry
1 teaspoon grated fresh ginger (or more, to taste)
4–8oz (115–225g) tofu, cut into cubes or slivers (optional)
2 tablespoons sesame seeds, for garnish

Place the stock in a large soup pot and bring to a simmer. Add the
Chinese cabbage and spring onions and simmer for 5 minutes, until the
cabbage is cooked through but still has some texture. Stir in the remaining ingredients, heat through and serve, garnishing each bowl with sesame
seeds.

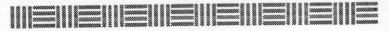

Sweet and Sour Cabbage Soup

serves 4–6

1 tablespoon safflower or sunflower oil
2 medium-sized onions, sliced
2 tablespoons sultanas
juice of 2 small or medium lemons (about 3fl. oz/90ml, or more, to taste)
2 tablespoons mild-flavoured honey
2 cloves garlic, finely chopped or put through a press
1 medium-sized cabbage, cored and cut into strips
salt, to taste
2 teaspoons paprika
1/4 teaspoon ground cloves
a 28oz (790g) tin tomatoes, with juice
1 1/2 pints (850ml) water or vegetable stock (see p. 80)
1–2 tablespoons soy sauce, to taste
2 slices dark rye or pumpernickel bread, diced
freshly ground black pepper, to taste
4–6 tablespoons natural low-fat yoghurt, for garnish

Heat the oil over a medium–low heat in a large, heavy-bottomed soup pot or casserole and add the onions. Sauté, stirring often, until the onions are soft: about 10 minutes.

Combine the sultanas, lemon juice and honey in a small bowl.

Add the garlic, cabbage and salt to the pot, stir together well, cover and sauté with the onions, stirring from time to time, for about 4 minutes.

Add the paprika, cloves and tomatoes and stir together well. Add the water or vegetable stock, soy sauce, more salt to taste, the raisin–lemon juice mixture and the bread. Bring to a simmer, cover and simmer for 45–60 minutes, stirring from time to time.

Taste and adjust the seasonings, adding freshly ground pepper to taste. Serve, garnishing each bowl with natural low-fat yoghurt.

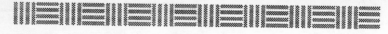

Hot and Sour Soup

serves 6

6 dried Chinese mushrooms
3 pints (2 litres) vegetable stock or chicken stock (see pp. 80 and 81)
1 tablespoon finely chopped fresh ginger
6 spring onions, sliced, white and green parts separated
8oz (225g) tofu, slivered
2 tablespoons dry sherry or Chinese rice wine
2fl. oz (60ml) cider vinegar or Chinese rice wine vinegar (or more, to taste)
2–3 tablespoons soy sauce (or more, to taste)
2 tablespoons cornflour or arrowroot
4 tablespoons water
2 eggs, beaten
1 large carrot, cut into 2-inch matchsticks
1 stick celery or bok choy (Chinese greens), cut into 2-inch matchsticks
3oz (85g) cucumber, cut into matchsticks
1/4–1/2 teaspoon freshly ground black pepper, to taste
2 tablespoons chopped fresh coriander

Before you begin cutting the vegetables, place the Chinese mushrooms in a small bowl. Bring 3/4 pint (425ml) of the stock to a boil and pour it over the mushrooms. Let them stand for 15 minutes, while you prepare the remaining ingredients.

Place the remaining stock in a large soup pot or casserole. Drain the mushrooms and retain the soaking liquid. Strain this through a cheese-cloth or coffee filter and add it to the stock. Rinse the mushrooms well, cut them into slivers and add them to the stock, along with the ginger and the white part of the green onions. Simmer for 5 minutes and add the tofu. Simmer for 5 more minutes and stir in the sherry, vinegar and soy sauce.

Dissolve the cornflour or arrowroot in the 4 tablespoons water. Stir this into the soup, bring to a gentle boil and simmer, stirring, until the soup thickens: about 3 minutes.

Drizzle the beaten eggs into the simmering soup, stirring with a fork or chopstick so that the eggs form shreds. Remove the soup from the heat and stir in the pepper. Taste and adjust the vinegar, soy sauce and pepper.

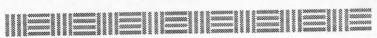

Distribute carrots, celery or bok choy, cucumber and the spring onion tops among the bowls and ladle in the soup. Sprinkle a little fresh coriander on each bowl and serve at once, passing additional pepper and vinegar so that people can adjust the hot and sour to their taste.

Miso Soup

serves 4–6

2½ pints (1.5 litres) water
1½oz (40g) kombu (kelp, available in wholefoods shops and Japanese markets – optional)
1 teaspoon grated or finely chopped fresh ginger
3–4 tablespoons miso, to taste (see note below)
4oz (115g) fresh mushrooms, sliced very thin
4 spring onions, sliced
4oz (115g) tofu, diced

Combine the kombu, if using, and water in a soup pot and heat slowly, so that the water takes 10 minutes to come to a simmer. Do not boil. When the water reaches the simmering point, remove the kombu. Omit this step if not using, and simply bring the water to a simmer. Add the ginger.
  Place the miso in a bowl and whisk in 4fl. oz (120ml) of the simmering water. Dissolve the miso and return to the pot. Keep at a bare simmer and add the mushrooms, tofu and spring onions. Heat through and serve.

Note   Miso is a paste made with fermented soy beans. A common ingredient in Japanese cuisine, it has a rich, savoury taste and is high in protein. It is also quite salty.

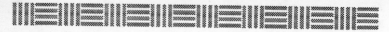

Tofu Noodle Soup

serves 4–6

2½ pints (1.5 litres) vegetable stock, garlic broth or chicken stock (see pp. 79–81)
8oz (225g) tofu, diced
8oz (225g) flat wholemeal noodles or spaghetti, or buckwheat noodles (soba)
2 eggs
juice of 1½ lemons
3 spring onions, green parts only, thinly sliced
freshly ground pepper, to taste

Simmer the stock and add the tofu. Simmer for about 10–15 minutes, until cooked through, then add the noodles or spaghetti. Simmer until the pasta is cooked *al dente* – still firm to the bite.

Beat the eggs in a bowl and add the lemon juice. Stir together, then ladle in some of the simmering stock. Stir this back into the soup, being careful not to boil it. Add freshly ground pepper to taste, and serve, topping each bowl with the sliced spring-onion tops.

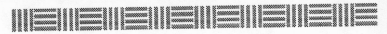

Blender Gazpacho

serves 6–8

This is great to have on hand in the refrigerator, not just for quick lunches but for snacks as well. Make a big bowl of it at the beginning of the week, and you'll be drinking salads all week long. It keeps well and is always refreshing.

1½lb (680g) ripe tomatoes, peeled
1–2 cloves garlic, to taste
½ onion, sliced
1 carrot, peeled and coarsely chopped
1 small cucumber, peeled and coarsely chopped
1 green pepper, seeded and coarsely chopped
2 sprigs fresh parsley
3–4 tablespoons fresh basil, if available
juice of 1–2 lemons, to taste
salt and freshly ground pepper, to taste
1¼–1½ pints (750–850ml) V-8 or tomato juice, depending on how thick
    you want it

Optional

4oz (115g) tofu, diced
a handful of alfalfa sprouts
2 tablespoons sunflower seeds
8fl.oz (225ml) natural low-fat yoghurt

Blend together all except the optional ingredients in a blender until smooth. Chill for several hours. Taste and adjust the seasonings.

Serve, using the optional ingredients as garnishes.

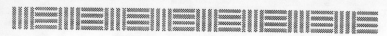

Chilled Yoghurt–Cucumber Soup

serves 4

1 large cucumber, peeled
2 cloves garlic, finely chopped or put through a press
1½ pints (850ml) natural low-fat yoghurt
4fl. oz (120ml) cold water
2 tablespoons chopped fresh mint
4–5 tablespoons fresh lemon juice
salt and freshly ground pepper, to taste
1 lemon, sliced paper thin, for garnish
1 additional tablespoon chopped mint, for garnish

If you are using a food processor, finely chop the cucumber and garlic together, using the pulse action, until the cucumber is minced very small, or like a coarse purée. Add the remaining ingredients and blend them together in the food processor until everything is just amalgamated – you don't want to lose the texture of the cucumber. Taste and adjust the seasonings. Chill for several hours, and serve with an ice cube in each bowl, garnished with fresh chopped mint and thin slices of lemon.

If you are mixing the soup by hand, chop the cucumber very fine, or grate it. Whisk together the yoghurt and water, and stir in the cucumber, garlic, mint, lemon juice, salt and pepper. Chill and serve as above.

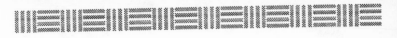

Main Dishes

After you peruse these recipes you will be convinced that a vegetarian weight-loss programme need not be a diet of deprivation. All kinds of cuisines are represented here: Italian, French, Indian and Middle Eastern, Chinese, Mexican and Tex-Mex.

You'll find that pasta is by no means excluded from this diet; it's just that the noodles are tossed with light vegetable-based sauces. Even lasagne has a place, filled with luscious tomato sauce, spinach and low-fat cottage cheese. Look for wholemeal pasta noodles, easy to find in wholefood shops and most supermarkets.

You could choose dinners from this chapter for a month and never repeat yourself, proof that a vegetarian diet need not be boring and predictable.

Some of the dishes here are very light, such as the chicken and fish dishes and vegetarian dishes like Chilled Tofu with Dipping Sauces (p. 131) or Broccoli Timbale (p. 127). Others are more substantial, stick-to-your-ribs dishes, like the Meatless Chilli on p. 158 and the Mushroom Risotto on p. 140.

You can make an entire meal out of these dishes, accompanying them with a salad or side-dish if you like. Or, with lighter soups or starter salads, they can be one course in a more elaborate meal. Let your appetite and the day's calorie intake be your guide. Bread on the side is optional, although I usually list it in the menus given at the end of the book. Limit your portion to one slice.

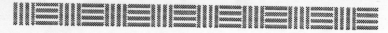

Grilled Salmon Steaks

serves 4

1 tablespoon safflower or sesame oil
1 tablespoon soy sauce
1 teaspoon freshly grated ginger (optional)
1 teaspoon mild-flavoured honey (optional)
four 4oz (115g) salmon steaks (about ¾ inch thick)

Combine the sesame or safflower oil, the soy sauce, ginger and honey. Marinate the salmon steaks in this mixture while you pre-heat the grill for 15 minutes.

Place the salmon 4 inches from the heat. Grill for 4–5 minutes on each side, basting once on each side. Serve at once, with wedges of lemon.

Fish Teriyaki

serves 4

1 lb (450g) fish fillets, such as sole, cod or whiting
1 tablespoon soy sauce
1 tablespoon dry sherry
1–2 teaspoons freshly grated ginger
juice of ½ lemon
1 tablespoon sesame oil

Mix together the soy sauce, sherry, ginger, lemon juice and sesame oil and place in a shallow baking dish. Lay the fish fillets in the dish, cover and refrigerate for at least 1 hour, turning once or twice.

Pre-heat the oven to 425°F/220°C/gas mark 7. Bake the fish for 8–12 minutes, until it is opaque and flakes easily with a fork. Serve hot.

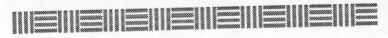

Steamed Fillets of Sole with Tomato Sauce

serves 4

1lb (450g) fillets of sole or Dover sole
salt and freshly ground pepper, to taste
juice of 1 lemon

For the tomato sauce

2 teaspoons olive oil
1–2 cloves garlic, finely chopped or put through a press
2lb (900g) tomatoes, tinned or fresh, seeded and chopped
1/2–1 teaspoon dried thyme, oregano or basil; or 1 tablespoon
    chopped fresh basil
salt and freshly ground pepper, to taste

First make the tomato sauce. Heat the olive oil in a heavy-bottomed or non-stick frying pan and sauté the garlic over a medium–low heat for 1–2 minutes, until golden. Add the tomatoes and bring to a simmer. Simmer over a medium–low heat, uncovered, for 30 minutes, stirring often. Season to taste with thyme, oregano or basil, and salt and freshly ground pepper. Mash the sauce with the back of a spoon and set it aside.

Now steam the fish. Salt and pepper the fillets lightly and sprinkle them with lemon juice. Arrange them on a steaming rack big enough for all the fish. Fill a large covered frying pan or saucepan big enough to accommodate the steamer with an inch or less of water (the water should not touch the bottom of the steamer when it boils). Bring the water to a boil, and place the steamer in the pan. Cover and steam for 5–7 minutes, until the fish is opaque and flakes easily with a fork. Remove the fish from the steamer and place it on a serving platter or on individual plates. Top with the tomato sauce, or place the sauce on the side, and serve at once.

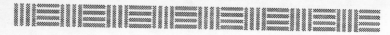

Sweet and Sour Prawns

serves 4–6

2 tablespoons cider or white wine vinegar
1 tablespoon mild-flavoured honey
1 tablespoon soy sauce
4 tablespoons water
1 tablespoon cornflour or arrowroot

For the prawns

1 tablespoon safflower or sunflower oil
4 spring onions, sliced
1 teaspoon grated fresh ginger, or ¼ teaspoon powdered
1 clove garlic, finely chopped or put through a press
1lb (450g) prawns, shelled and cleaned
10oz (285g) frozen peas, thawed; or fresh peas, steamed
    5–10 minutes, until tender and bright green

First mix together the ingredients for the sauce. Combine the vinegar, honey, soy sauce and water in a small bowl or measuring cup and stir in the cornflour or arrowroot. Set aside.

Heat the oil over a medium–high heat in a wok or large frying pan, preferably non-stick. Add the spring onions, grated or powdered ginger and garlic, and stir-fry for 1 minute. Add the prawns and stir-fry for 2 minutes, until pink and cooked through. Add the peas, toss together and stir in the sauce. Turn down the heat a little and cook, stirring until the prawns and vegetables are glazed. Serve immediately over hot cooked grains.

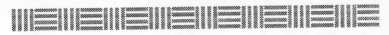

Fillets of Sole with Cucumbers and Dill

serves 4

Sole, cucumbers and dill go together nicely here. Dover sole or brill would also work.

1lb (450g) fillets of sole
olive oil for the baking dish
1 cucumber, peeled and cut in thin rounds
4 tablespoons chopped fresh dill
2 large cloves garlic, finely chopped or put through a press
2 shallots, finely chopped
juice of 2 lemons
salt and freshly ground pepper, to taste
4 tablespoons dry white wine (more if necessary)

Oil an attractive baking dish, large enough to accommodate the fillets in one layer. Lay half the sliced cucumbers over the bottom. Sprinkle with one third of the dill.

Rinse the sole fillets and pat dry. Score on the diagonal a few times with a sharp knife, and lay over the cucumbers. Lightly salt and pepper, and sprinkle on the garlic, shallot, another third of the dill and the lemon juice. Top with the remaining cucumbers. Cover with clingfilm and marinate in the refrigerator for one hour.

Preheat oven to 425°F/220°C/gas mark 6.

Sprinkle the remaining dill over the cucumbers. Pour on the white wine and make sure the entire surface of the baking dish is covered (add a little more if it isn't). Cover with lightly oiled foil or greaseproof paper and place in the oven. Bake for 10–15 minutes (5 minutes per ½ inch of thickness of the fish), until the fish is tender and flakes easily with a fork. Remove from the oven and serve from the baking dish, scooping up cucumbers from below and above the fish.

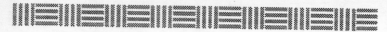

Fish au Gros Sel

serves 4

This isn't at all salty, despite the 5 pounds of salt. Because the skin and scales are left on the fish, none of the salt can penetrate. The salt becomes a hard shell, while the fish retains its juices and becomes succulent and tender.

one 2–2½ lb (900g–1.2kg) salmon, sea-bass or bream, cleaned but not scaled, head left on
5lbs (2.5kg) coarse sea salt
8 sprigs parsley
freshly ground pepper
lemon wedges for garnish

Preheat the oven to 425°F/220°C/gas mark 6.
Cover the bottom of a baking dish just large enough to accommodate the fish with a third of the coarse salt.
Stuff the cavity of the fish with the parsley and sprinkle with freshly ground pepper.
Place the fish on the salt and bury completely with the remaining salt. Make sure none of the skin is visible.
Bake in the hot oven for 25–30 minutes. Remove from the heat. You will hear the fish sizzling. Transfer the fish from the baking dish to a platter, shaking off the loose salt. A hard shell of salt will surround the fish. Gently break this, remove the fish and take off the skin, which will be salty. Fillet and serve at once, with lemon wedges.

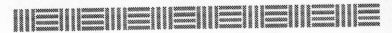

Grilled Sole

serves 2

You can't get much lighter or easier than this. For me a perfect meal, whether at home or at a restaurant, is a good salad and simply grilled very light fish like sole, accompanied with a green vegetable like spinach and maybe some steamed potatoes. This is especially good when cooked over a wood fire.

2 whole sole, about 10oz (285g) each, cleaned, skins removed
salt and freshly ground pepper
4 tablespoons freshly squeezed lemon juice
1 tablespoon olive oil
lemon wedges for garnish

Rinse the fish and pat dry. Season with salt and freshly ground pepper. Combine the lemon juice and olive oil, and marinate the fish in this for 20 minutes, turning once. Meanwhile prepare your grill.

Grill the fish for 4–5 minutes on each side and remove from the heat. Fillet the fish and serve at once, garnishing with lemon wedges.

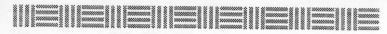

Steamed Cod Fillets with Tomato–Caper Sauce

serves 6

The sauce for this simple dish goes well with all kinds of fish.

For the sauce

1 tablespoon olive oil
1 small or ½ medium onion, finely chopped
8 tablespoons capers, rinsed and chopped in a food processor or mashed in a mortar with a pestle
4 cloves garlic, peeled and chopped (can be chopped or mashed along with the capers)
2½lbs (1.2kg) tomatoes, chopped
freshly ground pepper, to taste

For the fish

6 cod fillets
salt and freshly ground pepper, to taste

First make the sauce. Heat the olive oil in a large, heavy-bottomed frying pan and add the onion. Sauté for a few minutes and add the capers and garlic. Sauté, stirring, for 5 minutes, and add the tomatoes. Cook over a moderate heat, stirring occasionally, for 20–30 minutes. Season to taste with freshly ground pepper and set aside.

Steam the fillets. Measure the thickness of the fillets at the thickest point to determine the steaming time. Give 5 minutes per ½ inch of thickness. (Cod fillets are usually ¾–1 inch thick, sometimes a bit more.) Place on a rack or in a steamer over boiling water, cover and steam until the fish is opaque and flakes easily with a fork. Remove from the heat and place on a serving dish, or on individual plates. Spoon some of the sauce on top of the fish and more on the side, and serve.

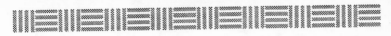

Cod Fillets with Tomato–Mint Sauce

serves 6

This sauce would go equally well with sole, whiting, bream and salmon.

For the sauce

2lbs (900g) tomatoes, peeled and seeded
1 small clove garlic
3 tablespoons chopped fresh mint
2 tablespoons balsamic vinegar
salt and freshly ground pepper, to taste

For the fish

1 1/2lbs (675g) cod fillets
salt and pepper, to taste
6 sprigs fresh mint
4 fl.oz (120ml) dry white wine
olive oil for the baking dish
fresh mint leaves for garnish

Preheat the oven to 425°F/220°C/gas mark 7. Brush a baking dish large enough for the fillets with olive oil.

Make the sauce. Blend together the tomatoes, garlic, mint and vinegar in a blender, or mash together in a mortar with a pestle until smooth. Add salt and freshly ground pepper to taste. This can also be prepared like Salsa Fresca (see p. 55), the ingredients finely chopped instead of blended together. The sauce can be chilled several hours, served at room temperature or heated through over medium–low heat in a saucepan.

Salt and pepper the fish and lay them side by side, on top of the sprigs of mint, in the baking dish. Add the wine and cover the dish with foil. Bake 10–15 minutes, until the fish is opaque and flakes easily with a fork. Transfer fish to a platter, top with the sauce, garnish with mint leaves and serve, putting additional sauce on the side.

Note This could also be served cold.

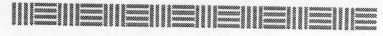

Fish Fillets Grilled in Foil with Garlic and Mushrooms

serves 4

These fillets should be eaten right from the foil packet so you don't lose any of the juice.

1lb (450g) of fillets of cod, bream, sea bass or other white-fleshed fish (should be four fillets)
1 tablespoon olive oil
salt and freshly ground pepper, to taste
8 large or 16 medium mushrooms, cleaned and sliced
5 cloves garlic, cut into lengthwise slivers
2 tablespoons dry white wine
2 lemons, cut into thin slices
4 large sprigs fresh rosemary, or 2 teaspoons dried
additional lemon, for garnish

Preheat the oven to 425°F/220°C/gas mark 7.

Cut squares of double thickness aluminium, each about twice the size of the fillets. Brush with olive oil.

Place a fillet on each square and sprinkle with salt and pepper. Top with the mushrooms and garlic slivers. Sprinkle with white wine and lay three or four slices of lemon over the mushrooms and garlic. Lay the rosemary over the lemon slices or sprinkle each fillet with dried rosemary. Bring the edges of the foil together over the fish and seal, crimping them together well so that no juice escapes.

Place the packets in a baking dish and bake in the hot oven for 10–15 minutes (check one after 10 minutes; the fish should be opaque and should flake easily). Serve at once, placing a packet on each plate and passing extra lemon wedges, as well as additional salt and pepper.

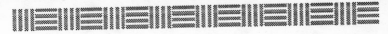

Grilled Chicken Breasts with Tarragon

serves 4

4 3–4oz (85–115g) chicken breasts, skin removed
1 teaspoon olive oil
salt and freshly ground pepper, to taste
juice of 1 lemon
1 large clove garlic, finely chopped or put through a press (optional)
1 tablespoon chopped fresh tarragon

Preheat the grill.

Brush the chicken breasts with olive oil, sprinkle with salt and freshly ground pepper, lemon juice and garlic (if using).

Grill for 5–7 minutes on each side, until cooked through. Sprinkle with the tarragon and serve.

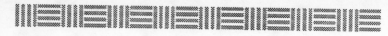

Chicken Breasts Baked in Foil

serves 4

These tangy chicken breasts are topped with garlic, lemon juice and zest, and baked in foil.

4 single chicken (or turkey) breasts, pounded to about ¼ inch thickness
salt and freshly ground pepper
1½ teaspoons olive oil for brushing chicken
2 large cloves garlic, finely chopped or put through a press
½ teaspoon chopped fresh or ¼ teaspoon dried rosemary
¼ teaspoon dried thyme
juice and zest of 1 lemon (yellow part only)

Preheat the oven to 375°F/190°C/gas mark 5.
    Sprinkle the pounded chicken lightly with salt and pepper. Cut 4 large double thicknesses of aluminium foil, large enough to fold loosely over each chicken breast. Brush with olive oil and set a chicken breast on each piece. Sprinkle the chicken breasts with garlic, salt and freshly ground pepper, rosemary, thyme, lemon juice and zest.
    Fold the foil over the chicken breasts, crimp the edges tightly together, and bake in the preheated oven for 20 minutes. Serve at once.

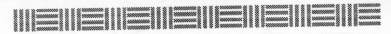

Chicken and Vegetable Curry

serves 4

1 tablespoon sunflower or safflower oil
10oz (285g) chicken breasts, diced
1 onion, sliced
1 clove garlic, finely chopped or put through a press
1 teaspoon grated fresh ginger
1–2 teaspoons curry powder (or more, to taste)
½–1 teaspoon ground cumin, to taste
1 large carrot, sliced
8oz (225g) shredded green or red cabbage
1 courgette, sliced
water
salt and freshly ground pepper, to taste
8fl. oz (225ml) natural low-fat yoghurt
1 teaspoon cornflour

Heat the oil in a non-stick frying pan or wok and sauté the diced chicken breast until cooked through. Remove from the heat and add the onion, garlic, ginger, cumin and curry powder. Sauté until the onion is tender, then add the carrot and a couple of tablespoonsful of water. Cook, stirring, for another 5 minutes, adding a little water if necessary, then add the courgette. Continue to cook for another 5–10 minutes, until the courgette is bright green and cooked through. Stir the chicken back into the pan and add a little salt and pepper.

Mix together the yoghurt and cornflour and stir it into the vegetable-and-chicken mixture. Taste and adjust the seasonings, adding more curry powder, cumin or salt if you wish. Heat through and serve over hot cooked grains, such as bulgur or brown rice.

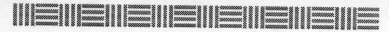

Grilled Chicken Breasts

serves 4

four 3–4oz (85–115g) chicken breasts, skins removed
1 teaspoon olive or safflower oil
juice of 1 lemon
1 large clove garlic, finely chopped or put through a press
1/2 teaspoon dried thyme
1/2 teaspoon paprika
freshly ground pepper, to taste
1/2 teaspoon cumin (optional)

Pre-heat the grill.

Brush the chicken breasts with olive or safflower oil, sprinkle with the lemon juice and top with the garlic and herbs. Add freshly ground pepper to taste.

Grill for 5–7 minutes on each side, until cooked through, and serve.

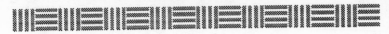

Stir-fried Chicken and Vegetables

serves 4

1 tablespoon safflower or sunflower oil
8oz (225g) chicken breasts, diced
1 onion, sliced
1 clove garlic, finely chopped or put through a press
1 teaspoon grated fresh ginger
1 large carrot, sliced
8oz (225g) cabbage or Chinese cabbage, shredded
1 tablespoon sesame or sunflower seeds
water, as needed
1 courgette, sliced, or 6oz (170g) broccoli florets
1 tomato, chopped
$\frac{1}{2}$ teaspoon dried basil
1–2 tablespoons soy sauce, to taste
1 teaspoon cider vinegar
1 teaspoon mild-flavoured honey
4 tablespoons water
1 tablespoon cornflour or arrowroot

Heat the oil in a non-stick frying pan or wok and sauté the diced chicken breasts over a medium–high heat until cooked through. Remove from the heat and add the onion, garlic and ginger to the pan. Sauté until the onion is tender, then add the carrot and a couple of tablespoons of water. Cook, stirring, for about 5 minutes, then add the cabbage and sesame or sunflower seeds. Cook, stirring, for another 5 minutes, adding a little water if necessary. Add the courgette or broccoli and sauté for another 5 minutes, then stir in the tomato, basil and the cooked chicken. Cover and simmer over a medium heat for 5 minutes. Meanwhile, mix together the soy sauce, vinegar, honey, water and cornflour or arrowroot in a small bowl. Stir into the chicken-and-vegetable mixture and continue to cook, stirring, until the chicken and vegetables are glazed. Remove from the heat and serve with hot cooked grains, such as brown rice, bulgur, millet or couscous.

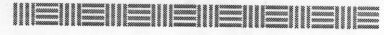

Rabbit Cooked in Chicken Stock and Wine with Fresh Peas

serves 6

Rabbit has no fat on it at all, so it's a perfect meal for the dieter. I like it cooked simply, in liquid, until it falls off the bone. Then it's very tender, with a marvellous flavour.

1 tablespoon olive oil
2 onions, finely chopped
4 cloves garlic, finely chopped or put through a press
one 3–4lb (1.5–2kg) rabbit, cut up
2 pints (1.2 litres) chicken stock (see p. 81)
½ pint (285ml) dry white wine
1 bay leaf
2 teaspoons dried thyme, more to taste
salt and freshly ground pepper, to taste
1lb (450g) fresh peas, shelled, or 6oz (170g) frozen, thawed

Heat the oil over medium heat in a large, heavy-bottomed casserole or stock pot. Add the onion and garlic and sauté until the onion is tender and beginning to colour. Add the rabbit, the chicken stock, wine, bay leaf, thyme, salt and pepper. Bring to a simmer, reduce heat, cover partially and simmer over very low heat for 1–2 hours, until the rabbit is tender and falls off the bone. Add the peas 5–10 minutes before serving and simmer until tender. Adjust seasonings and serve in wide soup bowls, accompanied with rice, pasta or potatoes.

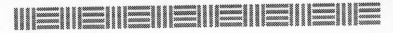

Piperade

serves 4

1 tablespoon olive oil
1 medium-sized onion, sliced thin
2 cloves garlic, finely chopped or put through a press
3 sweet green peppers, seeded and sliced into thin strips
2 sweet red peppers, seeded and sliced into thin strips
2 medium-sized ripe tomatoes, peeled, seeded and chopped
salt and freshly ground pepper, to taste
1/2 teaspoon dried oregano
1/2 teaspoon fresh or dried thyme
4 eggs
3 egg whites

Heat the oil in a large, heavy-bottomed, preferably non-stick frying pan and sauté the onion and garlic until the onion is tender. Add the green and red peppers and cook for about 10 minutes over a medium heat, stirring often. Add the tomatoes, salt, pepper, oregano and thyme, and mix together. Cover and cook over a low heat for 15–20 minutes, until the mixture is thick and fragrant.

Beat the eggs and egg whites together in a bowl and pour into the vegetable mixture. Stir constantly over a low heat, until the eggs set. Serve at once.

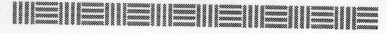

American Southern Spoonbread

serves 6

8fl. oz (225ml) water
¹/₂ teaspoon salt
6oz (170g) cornmeal
¹/₂ pint (285ml) skimmed milk
1 tablespoon low-fat margarine
3 eggs, separated
kernels from 1 ear of corn (optional)
1 hot green chilli pepper, finely chopped (optional)

Pre-heat the oven to 350°F/180°C/gas mark 4. Oil a 3-pint (2 litre) soufflé dish or baking dish, or a 10-inch cast-iron frying pan.

Bring the water to the boil in a 1¹/₂ pint (850ml) or larger heavy-bottomed saucepan. Add the salt and very slowly pour in the cornmeal, stirring continually with a long wooden spoon. Stir in the milk and cook over a very low heat or a double boiler, stirring continually, for 10–15 minutes, until you have a thick, smooth mixture. Remove from the heat and stir in the margarine. Stir in the egg yolks, one at a time.

Beat the egg whites until they form stiff peaks. Stir one quarter of them into the cornmeal mixture, then gently fold in the rest, along with the optional corn kernels and hot green chilli pepper.

Spoon the mixture into the prepared baking dish and bake for 30 minutes, until puffed and beginning to brown. Serve at once.

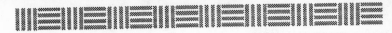

Broccoli Timbale

serves 6–8

1lb (450g) broccoli, broken into florets, the stems peeled and chopped
4 eggs
12fl. oz (340ml) skimmed milk
¼–½ teaspoon salt, to taste
½ teaspoon dried thyme
freshly ground pepper, to taste
2oz (55g) freshly grated Parmesan cheese
2 tablespoons chopped fresh parsley
sliced tomatoes and herbs, for garnish

Pre-heat the oven to 325°F/170°C/gas mark 3. Generously oil a 3-pint (2 litre) soufflé dish or mould. Steam the broccoli for 5 minutes and refresh it under cold water. Drain it and chop it fine (this can be done in a food processor). Set it aside.

Beat the eggs in a bowl. Heat the milk in a saucepan until the surface just begins to tremble. Remove from the heat, cool for a moment, then gradually whisk it into the eggs. Stir in the broccoli, the salt, thyme and freshly ground pepper, the Parmesan and the parsley. Pour into the prepared baking dish.

Put the dish in a pan of hot water and place in the oven. Bake for 1 hour, or until set and just beginning to brown. Remove from the oven, cool for 15 minutes or more, and carefully unmould on to a serving plate. Surround with sliced tomatoes and herbs, and serve.

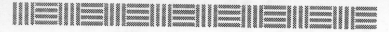

Mushroom Omelette

serves 4

1 tablespoon margarine, olive oil or sunflower oil
4oz (115g) mushrooms, sliced
1–2 cloves garlic (to taste), finely chopped or put through a press
1/4 teaspoon dried thyme
1/2 teaspoon soy sauce
freshly ground pepper, to taste
2 tablespoons chopped fresh parsley
4 eggs
6 egg whites

Heat the margarine or oil in a non-stick omelette pan and sauté the mushrooms with the garlic. When the mushrooms begin to be tender, add the thyme and soy sauce. Continue to sauté over a medium heat for about 5 minutes, until tender and aromatic. Add freshly ground pepper to taste and the parsley, and transfer to a bowl or plate.

Beat the eggs and egg whites together in a bowl. Heat the omelette pan and pour in the eggs. Swirl the pan to coat the surface evenly, and when a layer has cooked on the bottom, lift the edges with a spatula and tilt the pan so that the eggs can run underneath. Spread the mushrooms down the centre of the omelette and gently fold over. Cook for another minute or so, then turn on to a large serving plate. Divide into four portions and serve.

Note This can also be made as four individual omelettes.

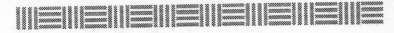

Mushroom Toasts

serves 4–6

This is inspired by a dish I ate while travelling through Belgium. It makes a comforting, filling supper.

1 tablespoon olive oil
8oz (225g) mushrooms, cleaned, trimmed and sliced
1–2 cloves garlic, finely chopped or put through a press
½ teaspoon dried thyme
½ teaspoon rosemary, crushed
1 teaspoon soy sauce
2 tablespoons dry white wine
freshly ground pepper, to taste
4–6 slices toasted wholemeal bread
2 tablespoons grated Gruyère

In a large, heavy-bottomed frying pan heat the oil and add the mushrooms and garlic. Sauté the mushrooms over a medium–high heat for about 10 minutes, stirring. Add the herbs, soy sauce and white wine and continue to sauté for another 5–10 minutes. Add freshly ground pepper to taste.

Heat the grill. Place the mushrooms over the toasted bread and sprinkle on the cheese. Place under the grill until the cheese just melts, and serve at once.

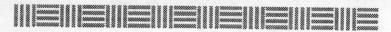

Baked Potatoes with Low-fat Toppings

serves 4

4 baking potatoes

Pre-heat the oven to 425°F/220°C/gas mark 7. Puncture the potato skins with a fork and bake for 40–60 minutes, until the potatoes are tender.

   Slit the potatoes open and cover with the topping of your choice (see below). You can also scoop out the potato and mash it with the topping, then return it to the skins and heat through.

Topping 1

4fl. oz (120ml) natural low-fat yoghurt
4oz (115g) low-fat cottage cheese
1 clove garlic
2 tablespoons chopped chives or spring-onion tops

Blend together the yoghurt, cottage cheese and garlic in a food processor or a blender. Stir in the chives or green onion tops.

Topping 2

4fl. oz (120ml) natural low-fat yoghurt
4oz (115g) low-fat cottage cheese
4 tablespoons chopped fresh parsley

Blend together the yoghurt and cottage cheese in a food processor or a blender and stir in the parsley.

Other Toppings

The same combination of yoghurt blended with cottage cheese – or use all yoghurt – seasoned with your choice of the following:

1 tablespoon tomato purée plus
   a pinch of cayenne
1–2 teaspoons Dijon mustard
1 teaspoon ground cumin

1 teaspoon curry powder
1 teaspoon caraway seeds
1 teaspoon soy sauce

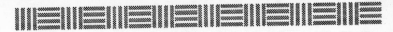

Chilled Tofu with Dipping Sauces

serves 4

1lb (450g) tofu, cut into 1-inch pieces
ice-cold water

Keep the tofu chilled in individual bowls of ice-cold water. Place the dipping sauce (see below and overleaf) in small bowls at each place.

Dipping Sauce 1

4fl. oz (120ml) water
4 tablespoons soy sauce, preferably tamari
3 tablespoons dry sherry or sake
1 tablespoon grated fresh ginger

Combine the water, soy sauce and sherry and bring to a simmer. Immediately remove from the heat and stir in the ginger. Serve warm or cool.

Dipping Sauce 2

2 tablespoons soy sauce, preferably tamari
3 tablespoons sake or dry sherry
3 tablespoons water
1 tablespoon mild-flavoured honey
1 tablespoon freshly grated ginger
2 cloves garlic, finely chopped or put through a press
2 teaspoons oriental sesame oil

Combine all the ingredients in a small bowl.

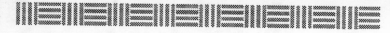

Dipping Sauce 3

2 tablespoons soy sauce, preferably tamari
1 teaspoon Japanese horseradish paste
pickled ginger

Combine the soy sauce and horseradish paste. Serve the pickled ginger on the side.

Grilled Tofu 'Cutlets'

serves 4

1 lb (450g) tofu, cut into four cakes
4 tablespoons water
4 tablespoons soy sauce
1 teaspoon mild-flavoured honey
1 teaspoon grated or finely chopped fresh ginger (optional)
1 tablespoon safflower or sunflower oil

To press the tofu. Wrap the tofu in a tea-towel with all the pieces in a single layer. Place on a baking sheet and set another baking sheet or cutting board on top. Place a weight, such as a saucepan full of water, on top of the cutting board or baking sheet and leave for 30 minutes or longer. The tofu will then be firm and compact.

Mix together the water, soy sauce, honey and ginger. With a skewer or fork, poke a few holes in each square of pressed tofu. Marinate the tofu in this mixture for at least 30 minutes.

Pre-heat the grill. Place the tofu on a baking sheet and brush with oil. Grill for 5 minutes on each side. Serve at once, with hot cooked grains and vegetables.

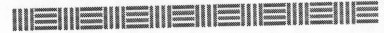

Stir-fried Tofu with Mangetouts

serves 4

8 small or 4 large Chinese black mushrooms
1 tablespoon safflower or sunflower oil
1 clove garlic, finely chopped or put through a press
2 teaspoons finely chopped fresh ginger
³/₄lb (340g) tofu, cut into 1-inch cubes
1 teaspoon soy sauce
½lb (225g) mangetouts, strings removed
3 spring onions, cut into 1-inch lengths

For the sauce
1 tablespoon cornflour or arrowroot
4 tablespoons water
1 tablespoon dry sherry
1 tablespoon oriental sesame oil
1 teaspoon mild-flavoured honey
1 teaspoon Pernod or other anise-flavoured liqueur
2 tablespoons soy sauce, preferably tamari

Place the mushrooms in a small bowl and pour on boiling water to cover. Allow to stand for 20–30 minutes, or until soft.

Combine the ingredients for the sauce and set aside.

When the mushrooms have softened, remove them from the soaking liquid, squeeze out excess water into the soaking liquid, and rinse the mushrooms thoroughly in cold water. Squeeze out excess water again and remove tough stems. Cut the caps into strips. Strain the soaking liquid through a strainer lined with kitchen paper or cheesecloth.

In a wok or a large non-stick frying pan, heat the safflower or sunflower oil over a medium heat and add the garlic and ginger. Sauté, stirring with a wooden spoon, for 10 seconds. Add the tofu and soy sauce, and stir-fry for about 1 minute. Add the mushrooms and mangetouts and stir-fry for another 2 minutes. Pour in the reserved mushroom liquid, cover and simmer for 5 minutes, or until the vegetables are crisp–tender. Add the spring onions. Stir the sauce mixture, making sure that the cornflour or arrowroot is dissolved, and add to the vegetables. Stir over a medium–high heat until thick. Remove from the heat and serve at once with hot cooked grains.

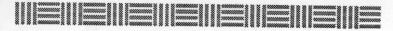

Stir-fried Tofu and Vegetables

serves 4

1 tablespoon safflower or sunflower oil
1 onion, sliced
1 clove garlic, finely chopped or put through a press
1 teaspoon grated fresh ginger
³/₄lb (340g) tofu, diced
1 tablespoon soy sauce
1 large carrot, sliced
water
¹/₂lb (225g) Chinese cabbage, shredded
2 tablespoons sesame or sunflower seeds
1 courgette, sliced; or 6oz (170g) broccoli florets
1 additional tablespoon soy sauce (or more, to taste)
1 teaspoon cider vinegar
1 teaspoon mild-flavoured honey
4 tablespoons water
1 tablespoon cornflour or arrowroot

Heat the oil in a non-stick frying pan or wok and sauté the onion, garlic and ginger until the onion is tender. Add the tofu and 1 tablespoon soy sauce and sauté, stirring, for 5 minutes. Add the carrot and a couple of tablespoons of water. Cook, stirring, for about 5 minutes, then add the cabbage and sesame or sunflower seeds. Cook, stirring, for another 5 minutes, adding a little more water if necessary. Add the courgette or broccoli and sauté for another 5 minutes. Add a little more water if necessary, cover and simmer over a medium heat for 5 minutes.

Meanwhile, mix together the soy sauce, vinegar, honey, 4 tablespoons water and cornflour or arrowroot in a small bowl. Stir this into the tofu–vegetable mixture and continue to cook, stirring, until the tofu and vegetables are glazed. Remove from the heat and serve with hot cooked grains, such as brown rice, bulgur, millet or couscous.

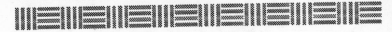

Curried Tofu and Vegetables

serves 6–8

2 tablespoons safflower or sunflower oil
1 teaspoon mustard seeds
1 teaspoon cumin seed, crushed
½ teaspoon turmeric
½ teaspoon chilli powder
2–3 teaspoons curry powder, to taste
1 medium-sized onion, sliced
1 clove garlic, finely chopped or put through a press
1 teaspoon finely chopped fresh ginger
½lb (225g) tofu, pressed if desired (see p. 132) and diced
½lb (225g) courgettes, sliced
1lb (450g) cauliflower, broken into florets and sliced
2 tablespoons raisins or currants
2fl. oz (60ml) water or vegetable stock (see p. 80)
salt and freshly ground pepper, to taste
1 tablespoon cornflour or arrowroot, dissolved in 1½ tablespoons water
8fl. oz (225ml) natural low-fat yoghurt
2 tablespoons chopped fresh coriander

Heat the oil in a large, heavy-bottomed non-stick frying pan, casserole or wok and add the spices, onion, garlic and ginger. Sauté until the onion is tender, then add the tofu. Sauté gently, stirring over a medium–low heat for 5 minutes, and add the courgettes and cauliflower. Cook, stirring, for 5 minutes. Add the raisins or currants and water or stock, cover and simmer for 5–10 minutes. Add salt and freshly ground pepper to taste, adjust the seasonings and stir in the dissolved cornflour or arrowroot. Cook, stirring, until the vegetables are glazed, then remove from the heat.

Transfer to a serving dish and stir in the yoghurt. Serve at once over hot cooked grains.

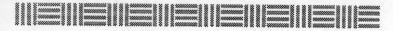

Crustless Tofu Quiche

serves 6

1 tablespoon safflower, sunflower or olive oil
2 cloves garlic, finely chopped or put through a press
1 small onion, chopped
1 ¼ lb (565g) tofu
4fl. oz (120ml) natural low-fat yoghurt
1 tablespoon wholemeal pastry flour
2 tablespoons soy sauce
1 teaspoon brewer's yeast; or ½ teaspoon Marmite
1 tablespoon light sesame tahini
1 teaspoon freshly grated ginger
juice of ½ lemon
½ teaspoon dried thyme
a pinch each of cayenne and nutmeg
freshly ground pepper, to taste

Pre-heat the oven to 350°F/180°C/gas mark 4.

Heat the oil in a frying pan and sauté the onion and garlic until the onion is tender. Set aside.

Combine the remaining ingredients in a blender or food processor and blend until completely smooth. Stir in the onion and garlic.

Oil a 2-pint (1.2 litre) baking dish, a loaf tin or a 9–10-inch *tarte* tin and pour in the tofu mixture. Smooth the top with a spatula and bake for 30–40 minutes, until it has set and the top is beginning to brown. Allow to sit for 10 minutes before serving, cut into squares or wedges.

This is good hot or cold, and will keep for several days in the refrigerator. It also makes a nice spread.

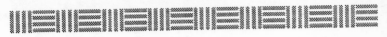

Tofu and Vegetable Skewers

serves 4

For the marinade
1 pint (570ml) natural low-fat yoghurt
1/2 onion, grated
2–3 cloves garlic (to taste), finely chopped or put through a press
1 tablespoon grated fresh ginger
2–3 teaspoons curry powder, to taste
1 teaspoon ground cumin
salt and freshly ground pepper, to taste
juice of 1 large lemon

For the tofu and vegetables
3/4lb (340g) firm tofu
1 tablespoon soy sauce
1 punnet cherry tomatoes, or 8 small tomatoes
1 green pepper, seeded and cut into quarters or eighths
1 sweet red pepper, seeded and cut into quarters or eighths
8oz (225g) large firm mushrooms, stems removed
1 medium-sized courgette, sliced 1/2 inch thick
1/2lb new potatoes, steamed until crisp–tender
soy sauce, for serving

Combine all the ingredients for the marinade in a large bowl.

Press the tofu according to the directions on p. 132 for 15–20 minutes, until firm but not dry. Cut into 1- or 2-inch squares and toss with the soy sauce.

Prepare the remaining vegetables and toss with the marinade. Cover with clingfilm and allow to marinate in the refrigerator for several hours, tossing at intervals to distribute the marinade evenly. Drain and reserve the marinade.

Prepare a barbecue or pre-heat your grill. Place the tofu and vegetables on skewers, alternating them to make a colourful arrangement. Roast over the barbecue or under the grill for about 20 minutes or a little longer, until the vegetables are cooked through and slightly charred, turning often to ensure even cooking.

Serve with hot cooked grains, with soy sauce and the marinade on the side.

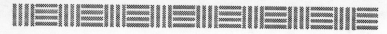

Vegetable Couscous

serves 6–8

¾lb (340g) chick peas, washed, picked over and soaked
2 tablespoons olive oil
1 large or 2 small onions, sliced
3–4 cloves garlic, finely chopped or put through a press
1 sweet green pepper, sliced
2 leeks, white parts only, cleaned and sliced
a 28oz (790g) tin tomatoes, without the liquid, coarsely chopped
3 pints (2 litres) water
1 bay leaf
1 fresh hot green chilli, seeded and sliced (optional)
salt and freshly ground pepper, to taste
½lb (225g) turnips, peeled and quartered, or cut into sixths if large
¾lb (340g) carrots, thickly sliced
cayenne, to taste
¾–1lb (340–450g) couscous
1lb (450g) courgettes, sliced
1 bunch fresh coriander, chopped

For garnish
harissa (see note below) or chilli paste (found in imported-food shops)
lemon wedges

Soak the chick peas overnight in three times their volume of water. Use bottled water if your tap water is hard. Drain.

Heat the olive oil in a large, heavy-bottomed soup pot or the bottom part of a *couscoussière*. Add the onion, half the garlic and the green pepper, and sauté until the onion begins to soften. Add the chick peas, leeks, tomatoes, the water, hot green chilli and bay leaf, and bring to the boil. Reduce the heat, cover and simmer for 1 hour. Add the remaining garlic, the carrots, turnips, and salt and freshly ground pepper to taste. Cover and simmer for another hour. Add cayenne to taste and adjust seasonings. At this point you can set the soup aside for several hours.

Thirty minutes before you wish to serve it, place the couscous in a large bowl or a casserole and gradually sprinkle on about ¾ pint (425ml) water.

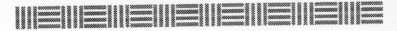

Let it sit for 15 minutes, stirring with a wooden spoon or between your palms and fingers every 5 minutes or more to prevent the couscous from lumping.

Meanwhile, bring the soup back to a simmer and add the courgettes. When the couscous is tender (add a little more water if you think it's necessary), add salt to taste, and heat it through in the top part of *couscoussière*, a strainer or steamer that fits tightly over your soup pot, or in a baking dish in a moderate oven. Simmer the soup for 10–15 minutes, until the courgettes are cooked through but still bright. Stir in the coriander.

To serve, spoon the couscous into warmed, wide, flat soup bowls and ladle on a generous helping of the soup. Pass lemon wedges and *harissa* (see note) or chilli paste, with a small bowl of broth so that people can dissolve the *harissa* in a spoonful before adding it to the couscous.

Note *Harissa* is a very hot chilli paste which can be found in imported-food shops. Indian chilli paste could be substituted.

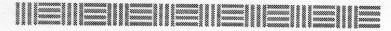

Mushroom Risotto

serves 4

1oz (30g) imported dried wild mushrooms, preferably *Boletus
    edulis* (porcini or *cèpes*)
³/₄ pint (425ml) boiling water
1¹/₂ pints (850ml) vegetable or chicken stock (see pp. 80 and 81)
1 tablespoon olive oil
2 shallots, or ¹/₂ small onion, chopped
3 garlic cloves, finely chopped or put through a press
8oz (225g) fresh cultivated or wild mushrooms, cleaned and sliced thick
10oz (285g) Italian Arborio rice
¹/₂ teaspoon dried thyme
¹/₄ teaspoon chopped dried rosemary, or ¹/₂–1 teaspoon chopped
    fresh rosemary
4fl. oz (120ml) dry white wine
1 tablespoon soy sauce
salt and freshly ground pepper, to taste
2 tablespoons chopped fresh parsley
4 tablespoons freshly grated Parmesan cheese

Place the dried mushrooms in a bowl and pour on boiling water to cover.
Let them sit for 30 minutes, while you prepare the remaining ingredients.

Drain the mushrooms and retain the soaking liquid. Strain this through
a sieve lined with paper towels and combine with the vegetable or
chicken stock. Bring this stock to a simmer in a saucepan.

Rinse the soaked mushrooms thoroughly, squeeze dry and chop.

Heat the oil in a large, heavy-bottomed, lidded saucepan or frying pan
and sauté the shallot or onion with the garlic until the onion is tender and
translucent. Add the fresh mushrooms and chopped dried mushrooms
and sauté over a medium heat, stirring, for 5 minutes. Add the rice, thyme
and rosemary and sauté with the mushrooms until all the grains are
coated with oil and the liquid from the mushrooms. Add the wine and soy
sauce and sauté, stirring, until the liquid is absorbed.

When the wine has just about evaporated, stir in a ladleful of the stock.
It should just cover the rice, and should bubble slowly, like the wine. Cook,
stirring constantly, until the stock is nearly absorbed. Add another ladleful
of the stock and continue to cook in this fashion, not too fast but not too

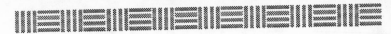

slow, adding more stock when the rice is almost dry. Continue to add stock, a ladleful at a time, and stir the rice, until the rice is cooked *al dente* – firm to the bite; this should take about 35 minutes in all. Add another ladleful of stock so that the rice is not completely dry, stir for a minute or two, add plenty of freshly ground pepper and remove from the heat.

Taste the rice and adjust the salt. Stir in the Parmesan cheese and the parsley, combine well and serve at once.

Brown Rice Risi e Bisi

serves 4

1¼ pints (750ml) vegetable stock (see p. 80)
1 tablespoon olive oil
1 small onion, chopped
2 large cloves garlic, finely chopped or put through a press
½lb (225g) brown rice, rinsed
4fl. oz (120ml) dry white wine
2lb (900g) fresh peas, shelled; or ¾lb (340g) thawed
    frozen peas
½ teaspoon dried thyme
salt and freshly ground pepper, to taste
3 tablespoons freshly grated Parmesan cheese
3 tablespoons chopped fresh parsley

Bring the stock to a simmer in a saucepan.

Heat the olive oil in a large, heavy-bottomed casserole and sauté the onion and garlic over a medium heat until the onion is translucent. Add the rice and sauté, stirring, for another 2–3 minutes, until the rice is coated with oil.

Add the white wine and cook, stirring, over a medium heat until the wine is just about absorbed. Pour in the simmering stock and bring to a second boil. Cover, reduce the heat and simmer for 35 minutes. Add the peas and the thyme and cook for another 10 minutes for fresh peas, 5 minutes for thawed frozen peas. Add more stock if the rice seems dry. Stir in the Parmesan and lots of freshly ground pepper. Add salt to taste, and the parsley. Serve at once.

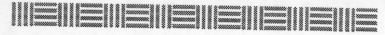

Aubergine Moussaka with Tofu Béchamel

serves 8–10

For the moussaka

2lb (900g) aubergines
1 tablespoon plus 1 teaspoon olive oil
2 additional tablespoons olive oil, safflower oil or butter
1 large onion, chopped
3 cloves garlic, finely chopped or put through a press
1 green pepper, cored, seeded and diced
1lb (450g) tomatoes, peeled, seeded and chopped
1/2–1 teaspoon dried thyme, to taste
1 teaspoon dried oregano, or more to taste
4oz (115g) bulgur, cooked (see p. 161)
1/2 teaspoon cinnamon
1/2 teaspoon allspice (or more, to taste)
1/2oz (15g) chopped fresh parsley
salt and freshly ground pepper, to taste
2oz (55g) freshly grated Parmesan cheese

For the tofu sauce

3/4lb (340g) tofu
1 tablespoon dark soy sauce, such as tamari or Kikkoman
1 1/2 tablespoons miso (see p. 105)
4fl. oz (120ml) natural low-fat yoghurt
2fl. oz (60ml) water
1 teaspoon finely chopped fresh ginger
1 tablespoon sesame tahini
1 tablespoon dry sherry
a pinch of freshly grated nutmeg
a small pinch of cayenne

Pre-heat the oven to 450°F/230°C/gas mark 8. Brush a large baking sheet with a teaspoon of olive oil.

Slice the aubergines in half lengthwise and score with a sharp knife, being careful not to cut through the skin. Place them cut-side down on the baking sheet and bake for 15–20 minutes in the pre-heated oven, until the skins begin to shrivel. Meanwhile, prepare the remaining ingredients.

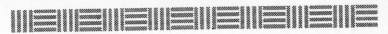

Remove the aubergines from the oven and, when they are cool enough to handle, scoop out the pulp and dice it. Reduce the oven heat to 350°F/180°C/gas mark 4.

Heat a large, heavy-bottomed frying pan or wok. Add the olive oil and sauté the onion with the garlic until the onion is tender. Add the green pepper and tomatoes and sauté for 3 minutes, stirring. Add the thyme, oregano and the diced aubergine and toss together (the aubergine will be very soft). Cover and simmer over a medium heat for 15 minutes, stirring from time to time. Uncover and stir in the bulgur, the cinnamon, allspice, parsley, salt and pepper to taste, and cook, stirring, for another 2 minutes. Taste, adjust the seasonings and remove from the heat.

Place all the ingredients for the tofu sauce in a blender or food processor and blend at high speed until completely smooth. Make sure you leave no gritty chunks.

Spread half the aubergine mixture over the bottom of an oiled 11x16-inch baking dish or a 6–7-pint casserole. Sprinkle one-third of the Parmesan cheese over this. Spread the remaining aubergine mixture over this and sprinkle on another third of the Parmesan. Mix the remaining Parmesan into the tofu sauce and spread in a thick layer over the top of the casserole.

Bake in the pre-heated oven for 25–30 minutes, until the top browns. Serve hot.

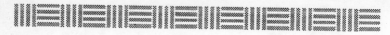

Pasta with Broccoli and Tomato Sauce

serves 6

2lb (900g) broccoli, broken into florets, stems peeled and chopped
1 tablespoon olive oil
2 large cloves garlic, finely chopped or put through a press
2lb (900g) ripe tomatoes, seeded and sliced
salt and freshly ground pepper, to taste
1 tablespoon raisins or currants
2 tablespoons chopped fresh parsley
1lb (450g) spiral pasta, preferably wholemeal

Steam the broccoli for about 10 minutes, until tender but still bright green. Refresh under cold water and set aside.

Heat the oil in a heavy-bottomed, preferably non-stick frying pan and sauté the garlic until golden. Add the tomatoes and salt to taste, and simmer for 15 minutes over a medium–high heat, uncovered, stirring occasionally. Add freshly ground pepper and the raisins or currants, and continue to simmer for another 5 minutes. Stir in the parsley and set aside.

Bring a large pan of water to the boil and add salt and the pasta. Cook *al dente* – firm to the bite – and drain. Toss with the sauce and serve at once.

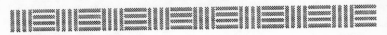

Pasta with Uncooked Tomatoes

serves 4–6

8 large ripe tomatoes, seeded and diced
1 tablespoon balsamic vinegar
3–4 tablespoons chopped fresh basil
3–4 tablespoons chopped fresh parsley
2 tablespoons capers, rinsed
1 clove garlic, finely chopped or put through a press
1 tablespoon olive oil
4 tablespoons freshly grated Parmesan cheese
salt and freshly ground pepper, to taste
³/₄lb (340g) fettucine or penne

Bring a large pan of water to the boil.

Meanwhile, toss the tomatoes, balsamic vinegar, basil, parsley, capers, garlic, olive oil and Parmesan cheese together in a bowl. Add salt and freshly ground pepper to taste.

When the water reaches a rolling boil, add a teaspoon of salt and a tablespoon of oil, then the pasta. Cook *al dente* – firm to the bite – drain and toss at once with the vegetable mixture. Serve immediately on warm plates.

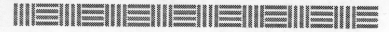

Pasta with Aubergine and Tomato Sauce

serves 4

1lb (450g) aubergines
1 tablespoon olive oil, plus 2 teaspoons for the baking sheet
4 cloves garlic (or more, to taste), finely chopped or put through a press
1 small onion, finely chopped
3lb (1.5kg) tomatoes, fresh or tinned
1 tablespoon tomato purée
salt and freshly ground pepper, to taste
a pinch of sugar
1–2 tablespoons chopped fresh basil
³/₄lb (340g) spaghetti, spiral pasta or penne
2 tablespoons freshly grated Parmesan cheese (optional)

Pre-heat the oven to 450°F/230°C/gas mark 8.

Cut the aubergines in half lengthwise and pierce each half on the cut side a few times with a sharp knife. Brush a baking sheet with olive oil and place the aubergines on it, cut-side down. Place in the oven and bake for 20–30 minutes, or until soft.

Meanwhile make the tomato sauce. In a heavy-bottomed casserole sauté the garlic and onion in the remaining tablespoon of olive oil over a low heat, until the onion is just turning gold. Add the tomatoes and tomato purée. Bring to a simmer. Add salt, pepper and a pinch of sugar, and simmer uncovered over a medium heat, stirring often, for 20 minutes. Adjust the seasonings, adding more garlic, salt or pepper if you wish.

When the aubergines are cool enough to handle, remove the skin and dice the pulp. Stir this into the tomato sauce and add the basil.

Bring a large pan of water to a rolling boil, and salt and cook the pasta *al dente* – firm to the bite. Drain, toss with the sauce and serve, passing the optional Parmesan cheese at the table.

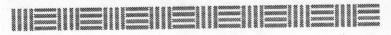

Pasta with Creamy Tomato Sauce

serves 4–6

The low-fat cottage cheese here makes this sauce seem rich. In fact it's high in protein and carbohydrates, but very low in fat.

2 teaspoons olive oil
1 onion, chopped
2–3 cloves garlic, finely chopped or put through a press
two 28oz (790g) tins tomatoes, drained and chopped, or 2lb (900g)
    fresh tomatoes, chopped
1–2 tablespoons tomato purée, to taste
1 teaspoon dried oregano
1 teaspoon dried basil
a pinch of cinnamon
salt and freshly ground pepper, to taste
1lb (450g) low-fat cottage cheese
1/2–3/4lb (225–340g) wholemeal spaghetti or other pasta
1oz (30g) freshly grated Parmesan cheese

Heat the oil in a heavy-bottomed casserole or wide, deep frying pan over a medium heat. Add the onion and one clove of the garlic and sauté until the onion is tender. Add the tomatoes and tomato purée and bring to a simmer. Add the remaining garlic and simmer over a low heat for 30 minutes. Add the herbs, salt and freshly ground pepper to taste, and then the cinnamon, and continue to simmer for another 15 minutes.

Remove from the heat and blend together with the cottage cheese in a food processor or a blender. Return to the pan and keep warm while you heat the water for the pasta.

Bring a large pan of water to a rolling boil, add a teaspoon of salt and the pasta. Cook *al dente* – firm to the bite: it will take 5–10 minutes, depending on the pasta. Drain, toss with the sauce and serve at once, or distribute the pasta among the plates and top each serving with the sauce. Pass the freshly grated Parmesan in a bowl.

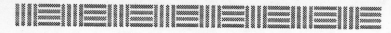

Spaghetti with Tofu–Tomato Sauce

serves 4–6

This spaghetti sauce proves that you don't have to have minced beef to make a hearty, meaty-tasting, high protein sauce for pasta. Those who are convinced they will never eat tofu won't even recognise this miracle food.

1 tablespoon olive oil
1 onion, chopped
2–4 cloves garlic (to taste), finely chopped or put through a press
½lb (225g) tofu
1–2 tablespoons soy sauce, to taste
3lb (1.5g) fresh tomatoes or two 28oz (790g) tins tomatoes, chopped
4 tablespoons tomato purée
salt, to taste
1 teaspoon dried oregano
½ teaspoon dried thyme
1–2 tablespoons chopped fresh basil, or 1 teaspoon dried basil
a pinch of cinnamon
freshly ground pepper, to taste
¾–1lb (340–450g) wholemeal spaghetti
4 tablespoons freshly grated Parmesan cheese

Heat the oil in a heavy-bottomed casserole or wide frying pan and sauté the onion with half the garlic until the onion is tender. Add the tofu and sauté, mashing with the back of a spoon, for about 5 minutes. Add the soy sauce and continue to sauté for another few minutes. Add the tomatoes and bring to a simmer. Add the tomato purée and salt, and continue to simmer over a low heat, covered, for 30 minutes. Stir in the remaining gar-lic, the oregano, thyme, basil and cinnamon, and continue to simmer for 15–30 minutes. Adjust seasonings, adding salt, garlic or herbs if you wish, and plenty of freshly ground pepper.

Bring a large pan of water to a rolling boil, add some salt and the pasta. Cook *al dente* – firm to the bite: this will take 5–10 minutes, depending on the pasta. Drain and toss immediately with the sauce, or distribute the pasta among warm plates and spoon the sauce on to each serving. Pass the Parmesan in a bowl and sprinkle on, to taste.

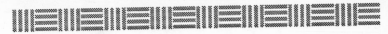

Spaghetti with Simple Tomato Sauce

serves 4

2 teaspoons olive oil
1½lb (680g) ripe tomatoes, peeled, seeded and chopped
1 clove garlic, finely chopped or put through a press
a tiny pinch of sugar
salt and freshly ground pepper, to taste
1 tablespoon slivered fresh basil
¾lb (340g) spaghetti

Heat the oil and add the tomatoes and garlic, sugar and salt. Cook over a medium heat for 20 minutes. Add the basil and adjust the seasonings.

Cook the spaghetti *al dente* – firm to the bite – in a large pan of boiling salted water. Drain, toss with the tomato sauce and serve.

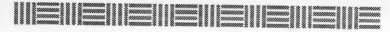

Spinach Lasagne

serves 6–8

You can use the tomato sauce below for this, or a good brand of commercial tomato sauce, which you can find in wholefood shops. You will need 1½ pints (850ml) of sauce.

For the tomato sauce
1 tablespoon olive oil
1 medium-sized onion, chopped
3 cloves garlic, finely chopped or put through a press
3lb (1.5kg) tomatoes, tinned or fresh, seeded and chopped
2 tablespoons tomato purée
salt, to taste
1 teaspoon dried oregano
1 teaspoon dried basil, or 1 tablespoon fresh basil
½ teaspoon dried thyme
a pinch of cinnamon
freshly ground pepper, to taste

For the rest of the lasagne
two 10oz (285g) packets frozen spinach, thawed
a handful chopped fresh parsley and/or basil (if available)
a pinch of nutmeg
1 egg
1lb (450g) low-fat cottage cheese
freshly ground pepper, to taste
6oz (170g) freshly grated Parmesan cheese
12 sheets wholemeal lasagne

First prepare the sauce. Heat the oil in a large, heavy-bottomed frying pan or casserole and sauté the onion and 2 cloves of the garlic until the onion is tender. Add the tomatoes, tomato purée and salt and bring to a simmer. Cover and simmer for 30 minutes. Add the remaining garlic, the oregano, basil and thyme, and simmer, covered, for another 30 minutes. Add the cinnamon and freshly ground pepper to taste, and set aside.

Squeeze excess moisture out of the spinach by wrapping it in a tea-towel and twisting it, then chop it fine. Beat the egg in a bowl and stir in

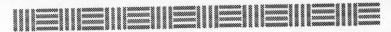

the cottage cheese, spinach, parsley and/or basil, and nutmeg and ground pepper.

Bring a large pan of water to a rolling boil, add a teaspoon of salt and cook the lasagne *al dente* – just firm to the bite: this will take 5–10 minutes, depending on the thickness of the lasagne. Drain and rinse under cold water. Lay the lasagne over the sides of the colander so that the water runs off as you assemble the dish.

Pre-heat the oven to 350°F/180°C/gas mark 4. Oil a 4–6-pint (3–4 litre) baking dish or casserole. Spread a very thin layer of the tomato sauce on the bottom of the dish and lay 4 sheets of lasagne across. Top the lasagne with one-third of the spinach–cottage cheese mixture, spreading it in an even layer over the lasagne. Spread one-third of the tomato sauce over this, and top with one-third of the Parmesan. Repeat the layers twice more: lasagne, spinach–cottage cheese mixture, tomato sauce, Parmesan.

Bake in the pre-heated oven for 40 minutes, until bubbling. Serve hot.

Note This can be assembled a couple of days in advance and kept in the refrigerator: allow an extra 10 minutes' baking time. It also freezes well. If it has been frozen, bake for 1 hour. The tomato sauce will keep for 3 days in the refrigerator, and can be frozen.

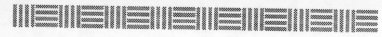

Homemade Pizza

serves 4–6

There is no reason why you shouldn't eat pizza, as long as it's not loaded with cheese and pepperoni or sausage, which are very high in fat. Almost all wholefood shops now carry frozen wholemeal pizza crusts, and there are good brands of tomato sauce available too. So in no time you can put together your own healthy versions, topped with whatever vegetables you like. Below are several ways to go about making pizzas, so that even those people who hate to cook won't be deprived of this treat.

Quick Wholemeal Pizza Crust

one 10-inch crust

8oz (225g) wholemeal or wholemeal pastry flour
1/2 teaspoon salt
1 teaspoon baking powder
1/2 teaspoon bicarbonate of soda
4fl. oz (120ml) water, plus 1–2 tablespoons, additional, as needed
2 tablespoons olive oil

Mix together the flour, salt, baking powder and bicarbonate of soda. Add the water and work in with your hands, then add the oil and work it in (this can also be done in an electric mixer or a food processor). The dough will be stiff and dry. Oil a 10-inch pie tin, pizza tin or quiche tin. Roll out the dough about 1/4 inch thick and line the tin. Since the dough is stiff, this will take some elbow grease. Just keep pounding down with the rolling pin and rolling out until you get a flat, round dough. Don't worry if it tears; you can always patch it together. Pinch a nice edge around the top and refrigerate it until ready to use. This can also be frozen.

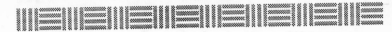

Yeasted Pizza Crust

one 10-inch crust

This is a delicious, crunchy crust with a slightly sour, earthy flavour that develops during the dough's long rising time. If you don't have this much time, double the quantity of yeast and allow the dough to rise for 2 hours.

1 scant teaspoon active dried yeast
5fl. oz (140ml) lukewarm water
1 tablespoon olive oil
½ teaspoon salt
4oz (115g) wholemeal pastry flour
4–5oz (115–140g) unbleached white flour

Dissolve the yeast in the water in a large bowl or in the bowl of your electric mixer and let it stand for 10 minutes.

Kneading the dough by hand. Add the olive oil and mix well. Combine the wholemeal flour and the salt and stir into the mixture. Begin adding the unbleached white flour and, as soon as you can, scrape the dough out of the bowl and knead it on a lightly floured surface for 10–15 minutes. The dough will be sticky, but keep flouring your hands and add only enough flour to prevent the dough sticking to the kneading surface.

Using an electric mixer. Add the olive oil and mix well. Combine the salt, the wholemeal flour and 4oz (115g) of the unbleached white flour, and add to the liquid all at once. Mix together using the mixing attachment, then change to the dough hook. Knead at low speed (1 on a Kenwood) for 2 minutes, then at medium speed (2 on a Kenwood) for 8 minutes. Add no more than 1oz (30g) of flour if the dough seems very sticky.

Shape the dough into a ball on a floured work surface and place it in an oiled bowl, seam-side up, then seam-side down. Cover and let it rise for 4–8 hours. If the dough doubles in size before this, punch it down. It needs the time to develop its full flavour.

To shape, oil your hands and the top of the dough. Punch down the dough and turn it out on to a floured work surface. Shape it into a ball and let it rest under a tea-towel for 30 minutes.

Oil a 12–15-inch pizza tin or baking sheet. Place the dough on the tin, then press and stretch with your hands, keeping them oiled so that the dough doesn't stick. Press out to a circle ⅛ inch thick, with a thick edge. Pinch the edges all the way around to make an attractive border. The dough can stand, covered with a tea-towel, for up to 1 hour before being topped and baked.

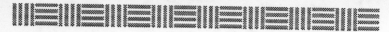

Tomato Sauce

1 tablespoon olive oil
2–3 cloves garlic, finely chopped or put through a press
2lb (900g) tomatoes, either fresh or tinned, seeded and chopped
2 tablespoons tomato purée (optional)
salt and freshly ground pepper, to taste
1 teaspoon dried oregano
1/2 teaspoon dried thyme
a pinch of cinnamon

Heat the oil in a heavy-bottomed frying pan or casserole and sauté the garlic for about 1 minute. Add the tomatoes and tomato purée and bring to a simmer. Add salt to taste and cook, uncovered, for about 30 minutes over a medium–low heat, stirring from time to time. Add the oregano and thyme and cook for another 15 minutes. Add a pinch of cinnamon and freshly ground pepper to taste. Taste and correct the seasonings, adding more salt, garlic or herbs if you wish. Set aside.

Toppings

Use any of these toppings, or a combination, with the tomato sauce above.

4 tablespoons grated Parmesan or Gruyère cheese
2oz (55g) skimmed-milk Mozzarella cheese, sliced
4oz (115g) tofu, sliced and sprinkled with soy sauce
2oz (55g) mushrooms, sliced and sautéed for 2 minutes in
   2 teaspoons olive oil
1 onion, sliced in rings
1 green pepper, sliced in rings
1 courgette, thinly sliced and sautéed for 2 minutes in 2 teaspoons
   olive oil

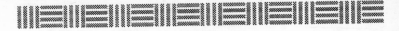

additional garlic, finely chopped or put through a press
1 sweet red pepper, seeded and sliced
2oz (55g) goat's cheese, thinly sliced
2 tablespoons capers, rinsed
freshly ground pepper

Make the pizza crust of your choice. If you are using the Quick Pizza Crust (see p. 152), pre-heat the oven to 450°F/230°C/gas mark 8. If you are using the Yeasted Pizza Crust (see p. 153), pre-heat the oven to 500°F/260°C/gas mark 10.

Spread the tomato sauce over the crust and top with other toppings of your choice. Bake for 15 minutes, or until the crust is brown and crisp.

Note You can make this pizza using bought, ready-made tomato sauce and crust, as long as they are reliable products (read the labels). Just assemble as instructed above and add the toppings of your choice. Bake as above.

All these pizzas can be frozen.

Pizza Sandwiches

See p. 49.

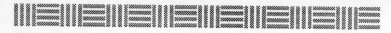

Black Beans

serves 6

1lb (450g) black beans, washed and picked over
1 tablespoon safflower or sunflower oil
1 large onion, chopped
4 large cloves garlic (or more, to taste), finely chopped or put through a
    press
2½ pints (1.5 litres) water
salt, to taste
3–4 tablespoons chopped fresh coriander

Wash the beans and carefully pick them over to make sure there are no
little pebbles disguising themselves as beans. Soak in three times their volume of water for several hours, or overnight. Use bottled water if your
tap water is very hard. Drain.

　　Heat the oil in a large, heavy-bottomed soup pot or casserole and add
the onion and 2 cloves of the garlic. Sauté until the onion is tender, then
add the drained beans and 2½ pints (1.5 litres) fresh water. Bring to a boil,
reduce the heat and cover. Simmer for 1 hour. Add the remaining garlic,
salt to taste and the fresh coriander. Continue to simmer for another
hour, until the beans are soft and the broth thick and aromatic. Correct
seasonings, adding more salt, garlic or coriander if you wish, and serve
with cornbread (see p. 26), corn tortillas, wholemeal bread or brown rice.

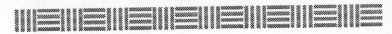

Black Bean Burritos

serves 6

These can be served hot or cold. If serving hot, serve the lettuce or alfalfa sprouts and tomatoes on the side.

6 wholemeal wheat flour tortillas or chapathis
³/₄lb (340g) cooked black beans (see p. 158)
1 teaspoon ground cumin
1 teaspoon chilli powder
1 teaspoon safflower or sunflower oil
2oz (55g) grated Cheddar cheese
2oz (55g) shredded lettuce or alfalfa sprouts
2–3 tomatoes, chopped

If you are preparing the *burritos* to be eaten hot, pre-heat the oven to 325°F/170°C/gas mark 3. Wrap the tortillas or chapathis in foil and place them in the oven while you prepare the beans.

Drain the beans, retaining about 4fl. oz (120ml) of their liquid. Purée coarsely, using the pulse action, in a food processor or blender, along with the cumin and chilli powder. Moisten with the liquid from the beans.

Heat the oil in a large non-stick frying pan and add the beans. Sauté, stirring, for about 10 minutes.

Remove the tortillas or chapathis from the oven and spread the re-fried beans down the centre. Top with the cheese and roll up. Heat in the oven for about 15–20 minutes, until the cheese melts. Serve with the chopped tomatoes and lettuce on the side.

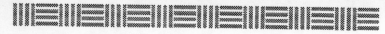

Meatless Chilli

serves 4

1 tablespoon safflower or sunflower oil
2 onions, chopped
4 large cloves garlic, finely chopped or put through a press
2 large carrots, chopped or grated
1 large green pepper, chopped
two 28oz (790g) tins tomatoes, drained and chopped; or
  3lb (1.5kg) fresh ripe tomatoes, chopped
4 tablespoons tomato purée
2 hot green chilli peppers, finely chopped
1 bay leaf
1 tablespoon chilli powder (or more, to taste)
1 tablespoon ground cumin (or more, to taste)
2 dried cayenne peppers, or ¼ teaspoon cayenne pepper
salt and freshly ground pepper, to taste
2 tins red kidney beans, with their liquid
1 teaspoon dried oregano

Heat the oil in a large, heavy-bottomed casserole or soup pot. Add the onions and half the garlic and sauté until the onion begins to soften. Add the carrots and green pepper, and continue to sauté for another 3–5 minutes, stirring all the time with a wooden spoon.

Add the tomatoes, tomato purée, chilli peppers, bay leaf and spices, and bring to a simmer. Add the remaining garlic. Reduce the heat, cover and simmer over a very low heat, stirring occasionally, for 30 minutes. Stir in the beans and oregano and continue to cook for another 30 minutes. Check from time to time to be sure that the chilli doesn't stick. Adjust seasonings, adding salt, pepper, garlic or cayenne to taste.

Serve with cornbread (see p. 26) or corn tortillas, or with wholemeal bread, and a big green salad.

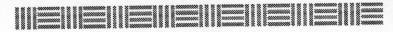

Soft Potato–Bean Tacos

12 tacos

Unlike traditional tacos, these are made with tortillas that have been heated but not fried, so they don't have nearly as much fat. They are called 'soft tacos' because the tortillas are not crisp. This makes them easier to eat than the usual kind. If you can't find fresh corn tortillas, make these with wholemeal chapathis.

1lb (450g) new or boiling potatoes, diced
1lb (450g) cooked black, kidney or borlotti beans (tinned may
   be used), with their liquid
1 teaspoon chilli powder
1 teaspoon ground cumin (or more, to taste)
1 teaspoon safflower or sunflower oil
1 small onion, sliced
12 corn tortillas or wholemeal chapathis
Salsa Fresca (see p. 55)

Steam the potatoes for 10 minutes, until crisp–tender. Set aside.

Place the beans and 2fl. oz (60ml) of their liquid, the chilli powder, and cumin in a food processor or blender and blend, using the pulse action, until just slightly puréed. They should still maintain some texture. You could also mash them in a mortar and pestle, or with a potato-masher.

Heat the oil in a heavy-bottomed, preferably non-stick frying pan and add the onion. Sauté, stirring over a medium–high heat, until tender. Add the potatoes and sauté over a medium–high heat until they begin to brown. Remove from the frying pan and add the beans, and a little more of their liquid if the frying pan is very dry. Sauté, stirring over a medium heat, for 5 minutes. Remove from the heat and clean the frying pan.

Heat the tortillas or chapathis in the frying pan, or steam above boiling water, until flexible and warm. Spread a heaped tablespoon of re-fried beans down the middle of each and top with a heaped tablespoon of the potato–onion mixture. Roll up the tortilla like an enchilada. Keep them warm in a medium oven while you prepare the rest of the tacos.

Serve warm, with Salsa Fresca.

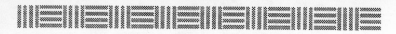

Grains, Pulses and Vegetable Side-dishes

Many of these delicious dishes made with grains and pulses can serve as main courses, often in combination but also by themselves, with vegetables on the side. They also make good side-dishes. For a light, nutritious supper you could serve two or more dishes in combination: Kasha with Vegetables (p. 173) along with Baked Tomatoes (p. 188), or Spiced Vegetables en Papillote (p. 189) along with Wild Rice and Mushroom Pilaf (p. 168), for example. I often make a very simple meal of the vegetable dishes alone – Baked Yams or Sweet Potatoes with Lime (p. 189) and Spicy Aubergines and Mangetouts with Miso (p. 178); Grilled Mushrooms (p. 181), Sautéed Red and Yellow Peppers (p. 185) and Saffron Millet (p. 170). I love to see the bright colours on my plate, and I love the combinations of flavours.

When cooking grains and beans, think about menus for the week. You might want to double the amount and use the extra for salads or stir-fries.

In addition to the vegetable dishes here, don't forget about unadorned steamed vegetables. Nothing can beat a serving of bright-green steamed broccoli, spinach or green beans. When my family lived in Connecticut, we used to make summer meals of steamed corn on the cob and vine-ripened tomatoes, when they were at their best. The corn needed no butter at all, it was so sweet. In fact most vegetables are so inherently good, they require no seasoning other than perhaps a little lemon juice or pepper.

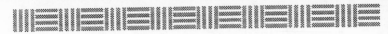

General Cooking Directions for Grains

6–8oz (170–225g) raw grain feeds four people.

Brown Rice, Barley

½lb (225g) serves 4

Use one part grain to two parts water (so for four people, use ½lb (225g) grain with ¾ pint (425ml) plus 2 tablespoons water). Combine the grain and water in a saucepan and bring to the boil. Add ¼ teaspoon salt, reduce the heat, cover and simmer for 35 minutes, until most of the liquid is absorbed. Remove the lid and if any liquid remains, cook uncovered for 5–10 minutes more, or until all the liquid has evaporated.

Bulgur

6oz (170g) serves 4

Use one part bulgur to two parts water. Place the bulgur in a bowl. Bring the water to a boil and pour it over the bulgur. Add ¼ teaspoon salt. Let it sit until the water is absorbed and the bulgur soft (about 20 minutes). Pour off excess water and fluff with forks.

Couscous

6oz (170g) serves 4

Use one part couscous, two parts water (tepid or hot). Place the couscous in a bowl, pour on the water and let it sit for 10–15 minutes. Fluff with forks.

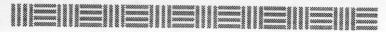

Kasha (Buckwheat Groats)

7oz (200g) serves 4

Use one part kasha, two parts water or stock. Have the stock simmering.

Method 1

Mix kasha with a beaten egg and sauté in a dry, heavy-bottomed saucepan or frying pan with a lid. Sauté the kasha until the grains are separate and begin to smell toasty. Add the simmering water or stock, cover and simmer for 20–30 minutes, until the kasha is tender but not mushy. Pour off any remaining stock.

Method 2

Heat 1 tablespoon sunflower or safflower oil in a heavy-bottomed saucepan or frying pan with a lid, and sauté the kasha until the grains begin to smell toasty. Add the simmering water or stock, cover and simmer for 20–30 minutes, until the kasha is tender but not mushy. Pour off any remaining stock.

To make a tastier kasha, begin by heating 1 tablespoon vegetable or safflower oil in the skillet and sautéing 1 chopped onion and 1 finely chopped clove of garlic until the onion is tender. Add the kasha and proceed as above.

Millet

7oz (200g) serves 4

Use one part millet to 2½ parts water. Heat 1 teaspoon safflower, sunflower or olive oil in a saucepan and sauté the millet until it begins to smell toasty and the grains are coated with oil (about 3–5 minutes). Add the water and bring to a boil. Add ¼ teaspoon salt, reduce the heat, cover and simmer for 35 minutes. Remove the lid and continue to simmer until the liquid has evaporated (up to 10 minutes more).

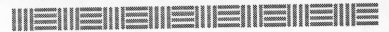

Wheatberries, Whole Rye, Triticale

½lb (225g) serves 4

Use one part grain, three parts water. Combine the grain and water and bring to the boil. Add ¼ teaspoon salt, reduce the heat, cover and simmer for 50 minutes to 1 hour. Remove from the heat and pour off any excess liquid.

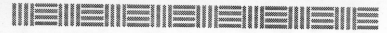

Wheatberry Pilaf with Mushrooms and Broccoli

serves 4–6

2½ pints (1.5 litres) vegetable stock, chicken stock (see pp. 80 and 81) or
  bouillon
1 tablespoon olive oil
3 cloves garlic, finely chopped or put through a press
½ medium-sized onion, finely chopped
8oz (225g) mushrooms, cleaned, trimmed and sliced
2 teaspoons soy sauce
½ teaspoon dried thyme
½ teaspoon crumbled dried rosemary
½lb (225g) whole wheatberries
4fl. oz (120ml) dry white wine
salt and freshly ground pepper, to taste
½lb (225g) broccoli florets
4 tablespoons freshly grated Parmesan cheese
2 tablespoons chopped fresh parsley

Have the stock simmering in a saucepan.

In a large, heavy-bottomed, lidded casserole heat the oil and sauté 1
clove of garlic and the onion until the onion begins to soften. Add the
mushrooms and remaining garlic, and continue to sauté, stirring, for
another 5 minutes. Add the soy sauce, thyme and rosemary, sauté for
another minute and add the wheatberries. Sauté, stirring, until the grains
begin to smell toasty: about 2 minutes. Add the wine and cook, stirring,
over a medium heat until the liquid has just about been absorbed.

Stir in the stock or *bouillon* and bring to the boil. Cover, reduce the heat
and simmer for 50 minutes, checking after 30 minutes to make sure that
there is still enough liquid. Add more if the mixture seems dry or near dry.

Add the broccoli, salt and freshly ground pepper to taste, and cover.
Cook for another 10 minutes. If a large amount of liquid remains in the
pan, pour some of it off. Stir in the Parmesan and parsley, and serve.

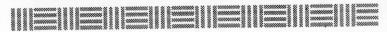

Courgette and Rice Terrine

Serves 6–8

1 tablespoon olive oil
1 onion, finely chopped
2lb (450g) courgettes, finely chopped
1–2 cloves garlic, (or more, to taste), finely chopped or put through a
  press
2 eggs
2oz (55g) Gruyère cheese, grated
1oz (30g) chopped fresh parsley
4oz (115g) short-grain brown or Italian Arborio rice, cooked
1/4–1/2 teaspoon dried thyme, to taste
salt and freshly ground pepper, to taste

Pre-heat the oven to 375°F/190°C/gas mark 5 and oil a non-stick loaf tin
or baking dish.

Heat 1 tablespoon of the olive oil in a large, heavy-bottomed frying pan
and sauté the onion until tender over a medium–low heat. Add the courgettes and the garlic, and sauté, stirring often, for 10 minutes over a low
heat. Remove from the heat.

Beat the eggs in a large bowl and stir in the cheese, parsley, rice, thyme
and sautéed vegetables. Add salt and freshly ground pepper to taste. Turn
into the prepared baking dish or tin. Bake for 40 minutes, until firm.
Remove from the heat. Serve hot, warm or cold, cut into slices or squares.

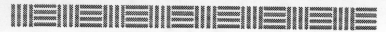

Italian Rice-stuffed Tomatoes

serves 4

4 large, firm tomatoes
salt and freshly ground pepper
6 heaped tablespoons Italian Arborio rice
4 cloves garlic, finely chopped or put through a press
12 leaves fresh basil, cut in slivers
3 tablespoons chopped fresh parsley
1/2 teaspoon dried oregano
3 tablespoons grated Parmesan cheese

Pre-heat the oven to 375°F/190°C/gas mark 5. Oil a baking dish.

Cut the tomatoes across the top, about one-third of the way down from the stems. Squeeze out the seeds and discard. Scoop out the pulp, chop and mix together with the rice, garlic, salt and pepper, the basil, parsley, oregano and Parmesan. Fill the tomatoes and replace the lid. Place in the baking dish, cover and bake for 1 hour (the rice will cook inside the tomatoes as they bake). Remove from the heat, allow to sit for a few minutes, or allow to cool completely, then serve.

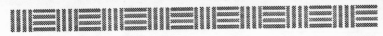

North Indian Pilaf

serves 6–8

This recipe, from my book *Spicy Vegetarian Feasts*, is adapted from Julie Sahni's 'Patiala Pilaf'.

14oz (395g) basmati rice
1 1/2 pints (850ml) cold water
1 tablespoon safflower or sunflower oil
1 onion, chopped
2 cloves garlic, finely chopped or put through a press
6 green cardamom pods
1 cinnamon stick, 3 inches long
8 whole cloves
1/2 teaspoon ground ginger
2 bay leaves
salt, to taste

Wash the rice thoroughly in several rinses of cold water. Soak in the 1 1/2 pints (850ml) cold water for 30 minutes. Drain the rice and retain the soaking liquid.

Heat the oil in a large, lidded frying pan or wok and sauté the onion until tender. Add the garlic and sauté for 1 minute, then add the spices and sauté for another 30 seconds, stirring.

Add the rice and more oil if necessary, and sauté over a moderate heat, stirring, until translucent and beginning to brown. Add the soaking liquid, salt to taste and bay leaves, bring to the boil, stirring, then reduce the heat and partially cover. Simmer for 10–12 minutes, until most of the water has evaporated and there are small steam holes covering the surface of the rice.

Now cover the rice tightly and place the pan or wok on a wok ring, a heat diffuser or asbestos pad. Turn the heat very low and continue to cook for 10 minutes, undisturbed. Turn off the heat and allow the rice to sit, undisturbed, for another 5 minutes. Turn it out on to a warm serving plate and accompany with a vegetable dish of your choice.

Note The whole spices are not meant to be eaten, but will do no harm if they are.

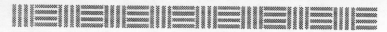

Wild Rice and Mushroom Pilaf

serves 4

6oz (170g) wild rice
1 pint (570ml) vegetable stock or chicken stock (see pp. 80 and 81)
1 tablespoon safflower or sunflower oil
1 small onion, chopped
2 cloves garlic (or more, to taste), finely chopped or put through a press
8oz (225g) mushrooms, cleaned, trimmed and sliced
1 tablespoon soy sauce
2 tablespoons dry sherry
1/2 teaspoon dried thyme
1/2 teaspoon crumbled dried rosemary
2–3 tablespoons chopped fresh parsley
salt and freshly ground pepper, to taste

Rinse the wild rice and set it aside. Bring the stock to the boil in a saucepan and add the rice. When the stock comes to a second boil, cover, reduce the heat and simmer for 40 minutes, or until the rice is tender. Drain off any remaining liquid and remove from the heat.

In a large, heavy-bottomed or non-stick frying pan, heat the oil and sauté the onion with 1 clove of the garlic over a medium heat, until the onion is tender. Add the mushrooms and remaining garlic and sauté, stirring, until the mushrooms begin to release their liquid. Add the soy sauce, sherry, thyme and rosemary, and stir together for a few minutes, until the mushrooms are cooked through and fragrant. Stir in the wild rice and heat through over a medium heat. Add the parsley, and salt and freshly ground pepper to taste, and serve.

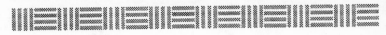

Bulgur Pilaf

serves 4

Double the quantity of this savoury pilaf and make Bulgur Pilaf Salad for tomorrow's lunch.

1 tablespoon olive, sunflower or safflower oil
1 medium-sized onion, chopped
1 large clove garlic, finely chopped or put through a press
2oz (55g) mushrooms, sliced
2 tablespoons dry white wine
6oz (170g) bulgur
1/4 teaspoon salt
3/4 pint (425ml) boiling water
soy sauce and freshly ground pepper, to taste

Heat the oil in a lidded, non-stick frying pan, a wok or a heavy-bottomed casserole and add the onion and garlic. Sauté until the onion is tender, then add the mushrooms. Continue to sauté for another 5 minutes, until the mushrooms begin to release their liquid. Add the wine and sauté for another 5 minutes, stirring, until the mushrooms are tender. Add the bulgur and salt, stir together well, then pour in the boiling water. Cover and turn off the heat. Allow to sit for 20–30 minutes without lifting the lid. Then check to see that the bulgur is soft (it should be, but if it isn't, pour on some more boiling water and wait for another 15 minutes). Fluff with forks and add soy sauce and freshly ground pepper to taste. Serve hot.

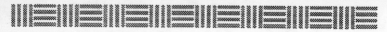

Saffron Millet

serves 4

1 pint (570ml) vegetable stock (see p. 80) or water
1 tablespoon safflower or sunflower oil
1/2lb (225g) millet
1/2 teaspoon crushed saffron threads
1/4 teaspoon salt
1 tablespoon lemon juice

In a small saucepan, bring the stock or water to a boil.

In a medium-sized, heavy-bottomed saucepan, heat the oil over a medium heat and sauté the millet for about 2 minutes, until it begins to smell toasty. Pour in the stock or water and bring to the boil. Stir in the saffron, salt and lemon juice. Reduce the heat, cover and cook for 35–40 minutes, or until the liquid is absorbed. Keep covered until ready to serve.

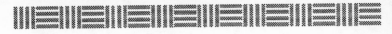

Lentil and Bulgur Pilaf

serves 6–8

½lb (225g) lentils, washed and picked over
2½ pints (1.5 litres) water
2 cloves garlic, finely chopped or put through a press
1 bay leaf
1 teaspoon ground cumin
a pinch of cayenne
salt and freshly ground pepper
6oz (170g) bulgur
1 tablespoon olive oil
1 large onion, chopped
2 tablespoons chopped fresh parsley or coriander
4fl. oz (120ml) natural low-fat yoghurt, for topping

Soak the lentils in the water in a large casserole for 1 hour. Add the garlic, bay leaf and cumin and bring to the boil. Reduce the heat and simmer for 20–30 minutes, until tender. Towards the end of cooking, add the cayenne, and salt and freshly ground pepper to taste.

Stir the bulgur into the lentils (there should be plenty of liquid left), cover and turn off the heat. Allow to sit for 20–30 minutes, until the bulgur has absorbed the liquid from the lentils and become tender.

Meanwhile, sauté the onion in the olive oil over a low heat in a non-stick frying pan, until almost caramelised.

Taste the bulgur and lentils and adjust the seasonings. Transfer to a serving plate and sprinkle on the onion and parsley or coriander. Serve, topped with natural low-fat yoghurt.

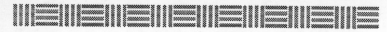

Middle Eastern Lentils with Vegetables

serves 6–8

½lb (225g) brown or green lentils, washed and picked over
1½ pints (850ml) water
1 bay leaf
3 sticks celery
2 carrots, sliced
½lb (225g) leeks, trimmed, cleaned and sliced
1lb (450g) tomatoes, skinned and chopped
salt and freshly ground pepper, to taste
1 teaspoon crushed coriander seeds
1½ teaspoons crushed cumin
a pinch of cayenne
1 tablespoon olive oil
1 large onion, sliced thin
3–4 large cloves garlic, finely chopped or put through a press
3–4 tablespoons chopped fresh coriander
juice of 1 lemon

Soak the lentils in the water in a large casserole for 1 hour. Bring to the boil, add the bay leaf, cover and simmer for 20 minutes, until just about tender. Add the celery, carrots, leeks, tomatoes, salt and pepper to taste, the crushed coriander seeds, cumin and cayenne, and continue to simmer for another 20—25 minutes, until the vegetables are tender and the liquid just about absorbed.

Meanwhile, heat the olive oil in a frying pan and sauté the onion until it is golden. Add the garlic, cook for another few minutes, stirring, then stir this into the lentils. Taste and adjust the seasonings. Transfer to a serving dish and sprinkle with the chopped coriander and lemon juice, or sprinkle with the coriander and lemon juice and serve from the casserole.

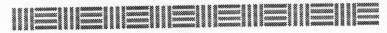

Kasha with Vegetables

serves 6

³/₄lb (340g) kasha (buckweat groats)
I egg, beaten
I¹/₄ pints (710ml) vegetable stock, chicken stock (see pp. 80 and 81) or
  bouillon
I tablespoon safflower or sunflower oil
I small onion, chopped
I clove garlic, finely chopped or put through a press
4oz (115g) mushrooms, cleaned, trimmed and sliced
soy sauce, to taste (optional)
I tablespoon dry sherry
I medium-sized carrot, chopped
I stick celery, chopped
salt and freshly ground pepper, to taste
4fl. oz (120ml) natural low-fat yoghurt, for garnish

Toss together the kasha and beaten egg in a bowl until all the grains are coated with egg.

Have the stock simmering in a saucepan.

Heat a wide, heavy-bottomed or non-stick frying pan or saucepan over a medium heat and add the kasha. Stir over the heat until all the egg has been absorbed by the grains and they are beginning to smell toasty. Pour in the stock, bring to the boil, reduce the heat, cover and simmer for 20 minutes, or until the grains are tender but not mushy.

Meanwhile, heat the oil in another frying pan and sauté the onion and garlic over a medium heat until the onion is tender. Add the mushrooms and sauté for about 5 minutes, stirring. Add the soy sauce and sherry, the carrot and celery, and sauté, stirring, for 5–10 minutes, or until the vegetables are tender and fragrant.

When the kasha is tender, drain off any excess water and add the grains to the vegetables. Stir together, adjust the salt and pepper, and heat through. Serve hot, topping each serving with a dollop of natural low-fat yoghurt.

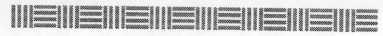

Savoury Haricot Beans

serves 4

½lb (225g) dried haricot beans, or two 14oz (395g) tins
2 tablespoons olive oil, in all (if using dried beans)
1 onion, chopped
2 cloves garlic, finely chopped or put through a press
2 pints (1.2 litres) water
1 bay leaf
salt, to taste
1lb (450g) tomatoes, fresh or tinned, skinned and chopped
¼ teaspoon dried thyme, or ½–1 teaspoon fresh thyme
1–2 tablespoons chopped fresh basil
freshly ground pepper, to taste
lemon juice (optional)

If using dried haricot beans

Pick over and wash the beans and soak them in 2 pints (1.2 litres) water overnight or for several hours (use bottled water if your tap water is hard). Drain.

Heat 1 tablespoon of the oil in a large, heavy-bottomed saucepan or casserole and sauté the onion and 1 clove of the garlic until the onion is tender. Add the beans, along with 1½ pints (850ml) fresh water, and the bay leaf. Bring to the boil, reduce the heat, cover and simmer for 1½ hours, or until the beans are tender. Add salt to taste, remove the bay leaf, drain the beans and retain the cooking liquid.

Heat the remaining oil in a wide, heavy-bottomed frying pan or casserole and sauté the additional garlic for 1 minute over a medium heat. Add the tomatoes and thyme, salt to taste and bring to a simmer. Simmer for 10 minutes, then add the beans and 4fl. oz (120ml) of their liquid, and the basil. Cover and simmer for another 15–20 minutes. Adjust the seasonings, adding freshly ground pepper to taste and lemon juice if you wish. Remove from the heat and serve.

If using tinned beans

Drain the tinned beans and retain the liquid, adding enough water to measure 4fl. oz (120ml).

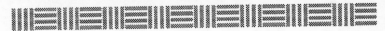

Heat 1 tablespoon of olive oil over a medium heat in a wide, heavy-bottomed frying pan or casserole and sauté the onion with 2 cloves garlic until the onion is tender. Add the tomatoes and thyme, and proceed as above.

Greek-style Haricots

serves 6

1 tablespoon olive oil
1 onion, chopped
4–6 cloves garlic, finely chopped or put through a press
1lb (450g) haricot beans, washed, picked over and soaked
2½ pints (1.5 litres) water
1 bay leaf
1 teaspoon dried oregano
2 tablespoons tomato purée
salt and freshly ground pepper, to taste
juice of 1 large lemon (or more, to taste)
½oz (15g) chopped fresh parsley
½ red onion, finely chopped

Heat the olive oil in a large soup pot and sauté the onion over a medium heat until it begins to soften. Add the garlic and sauté for a few minutes longer.

Drain the beans and add them to the pan, along with the water, bay leaf, oregano and tomato purée. Bring to the boil, cover, reduce the heat and simmer for 1–2 hours, until the beans are tender. Season to taste with salt and freshly ground pepper.

Remove the beans from the heat and add the lemon juice, parsley and chopped red onion. Adjust the seasonings, adding more garlic, salt and pepper if you wish, and serve.

Note This can also be served cold. In that case, allow the beans to cool before adding the lemon juice, parsley and onion. Chill the beans and add the last three ingredients shortly before serving.

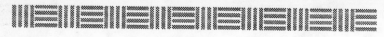

Chick Peas with Spinach

serves 6

½lb (225g) dried chick peas, washed, picked over and soaked
2½ pints (1.5 litres) water
1lb (450g) fresh spinach, stemmed and washed
1 tablespoon olive oil
1 teaspoon crushed coriander seeds
salt and freshly ground pepper
juice of ½ lemon
½ pint (285ml) natural low-fat yoghurt
1 teaspoon dried mint, or 2 teaspoons chopped fresh mint
2 large cloves garlic, crushed or put through a press
paprika, to taste

Soak the chick peas for several hours, drain them and combine them with the water in a large pan. Bring to the boil, reduce the heat, cover and simmer for 1½–2 hours, until tender. Add salt to taste. Drain and retain 6fl. oz (180ml) of the cooking liquid.

Wash the spinach but don't dry it, and chop the leaves finely.

Heat the olive oil and add the coriander seeds. Sauté for about 30 seconds. Add the spinach and cook over a medium–high heat for about 5 minutes. Add the chick peas and about 4fl. oz (120ml) of their liquid, season with a little salt and pepper, and simmer, uncovered, for 5–10 minutes, until the liquid is absorbed. Stir in the lemon juice and transfer to a serving dish.

Stir the crushed garlic into the yoghurt, then add the mint, and salt and pepper to taste. Pour over the chick peas and spinach, and sprinkle with paprika. Serve warm or chilled.

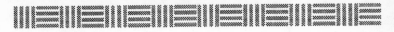

Black-eyed Beans with Tomatoes and Herbs

serves 6

1 tablespoon olive, safflower or sunflower oil
1 medium-sized or large onion, chopped
3 cloves garlic (or more, to taste), finely chopped or put through a press
1lb (450g) black-eyed beans
2¹/₂ pints (1.5 litres) water
1 bay leaf
1lb (450g) tomatoes, chopped
salt and freshly ground pepper, to taste
1–2 tablespoons chopped fresh basil, parsley or coriander

Heat the oil in a large, heavy-bottomed saucepan and sauté the onion with 1 clove of the garlic until the onion is tender. Add the black-eyed beans, the water and the bay leaf and bring to the boil. Cover, reduce the heat and simmer for 30 minutes. Add the remaining garlic, the tomatoes, and salt and freshly ground pepper to taste, and simmer for another 15–30 minutes, until the beans are tender but not mushy. Stir in the fresh herbs shortly before serving. Serve hot.

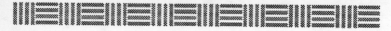

Steamed Artichokes with Low-fat Yoghurt Dressing

serves 4

This could be eaten as a starter, as a side-dish, or as a very light lunch or supper.

4 artichokes
1 recipe Low-fat Yoghurt Dressing (see p. 53)

Wash the artichokes and trim the stems. Cut off the very tops, then trim the leaves with scissors. Place on a steamer above boiling water, cover and steam for 45 minutes, or until the leaves pull away easily.

Meanwhile make the yoghurt dressing. Serve the artichokes hot, at room temperature or chilled, and dip the leaves in the dressing.

Spicy Aubergines and Mangetouts with Miso

serves 6

1/2lb (225g) mangetouts, trimmed
1lb (450g) aubergines, peeled and diced
2 tablespoons dark miso (see p. 105)
3 tablespoons water
1 teaspoon mild-flavoured honey
1 teaspoon sesame oil
1 tablespoon safflower or sunflower oil
2 cloves garlic, finely chopped or put through a press
2 teaspoons finely chopped or grated fresh ginger
8 spring onions, both white parts and green, sliced
1/2 teaspoon red chilli pepper flakes; or 1 small dried red chilli pepper, crumbled, seeds removed

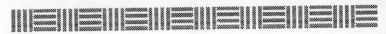

Steam the mangetouts for 5–10 minutes, to taste, refresh under cold water and set aside. Steam the aubergines for 10–15 minutes, until just about tender. Set aside.

In a small bowl mix together the miso, water, honey and sesame oil. Set aside.

Heat the oil in a wok or a large, heavy-bottomed frying pan and add the aubergines. Sauté for 5 minutes, stirring. Add the garlic and ginger and sauté for another 10 minutes, stirring. Add the miso mixture and continue to stir-fry for another 3–5 minutes, then add the spring onions and chilli flakes or crumbled chilli and cook, stirring, until the onions and aubergines are tender. If necessary, add 2–3 tablespoons water. Add the mangetouts, toss together well, heat through and serve over hot cooked grains.

Courgettes with Tomatoes and Basil

serves 4–6

1 tablespoon olive oil
1½lb (680g) courgettes, sliced about ¼ inch thick
2 cloves garlic, finely chopped or put through a press
1lb (450g) tomatoes, chopped
salt and freshly ground pepper, to taste
1 tablespoon chopped fresh basil

Heat the olive oil in a wide, heavy-bottomed frying pan and sauté the courgettes with the garlic over a medium heat for 5 minutes. Add the tomatoes, salt and pepper, and bring to a simmer. Simmer over a medium–low heat, stirring from time to time, for 15–20 minutes. Add the basil, correct the seasonings and serve.

You could also serve this cold, with a little lemon juice squeezed over the top.

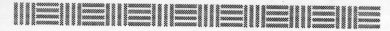

Cucumbers Simmered in White Wine

serves 4–6

1 tablespoon olive oil
2 tablespoons chopped onion or shallot
½–1 teaspoon ground cumin, to taste
½–1 teaspoon curry powder, to taste
2 large or 4 small cucumbers, peeled and sliced
juice of ½ lemon
4fl. oz (120ml) dry white wine
salt and freshly ground pepper, to taste
2 tablespoons chopped fresh parsley or coriander

Heat the oil in a heavy-bottomed, lidded frying pan or casserole over a medium heat, and sauté the onion until it begins to soften. Add the cumin and curry powder, stir together and add the cucumber. Sauté, stirring, for a minute or two, then add the lemon juice and white wine. Bring to a simmer, reduce the heat, cover and simmer for 20 minutes.

Uncover and turn up the heat. Boil off most of the wine, stirring. Add salt and freshly ground pepper to taste, toss with the parsley or coriander and serve, or chill and serve cold.

Steamed Greens with Vinegar or Lemon Juice

serves 4–6

2lb (900g) kale or collard, mustard or turnip greens, stems trimmed
  away, washed well and coarsely chopped
1 tablespoon olive oil
1 clove garlic, finely chopped or put through a press
1–2 tablespoons white wine vinegar or lemon juice, to taste
freshly ground pepper, to taste

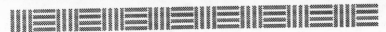

Wash the greens, and heat a wide, heavy frying-pan. Add the greens and steam them in their own liquid, stirring, for about 5 minutes, or until wilted. Remove from the pan and let the liquid in the pan evaporate over a medium heat.

Heat the olive oil in the pan and add the garlic. Sauté for a minute or so, then add the greens. Sauté, stirring, for about 3 minutes, then stir in the vinegar or lemon juice and freshly ground pepper to taste. Heat through and serve. (This can also be done in advance and reheated.)

Grilled Mushrooms

serves 4

1lb (450g) mushrooms, cleaned and stems removed
1 tablespoon olive oil
3 cloves garlic, cut in thin slivers
$1/2$ teaspoon crumbled dried rosemary
$1/4$ teaspoon dried thyme
salt and freshly ground pepper, to taste

Pre-heat the grill. Oil a baking sheet.

Place the mushrooms on the baking sheet, rounded-side down. Drizzle on the olive oil and sprinkle on the garlic, thyme, rosemary, salt and pepper.

Place under the grill, about 4 inches away, and cook for 10–15 minutes, basting every 5 minutes with the juices released by the mushrooms. Turn the mushrooms over during the last 5 minutes. Remove from the heat and serve as a side-dish or first course.

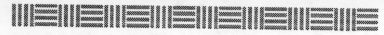

Spicy Green Beans

serves 4–6

1lb (450g) green beans, ends trimmed
3 tablespoons natural low-fat yoghurt
1 hot fresh green chilli, thinly sliced
1 teaspoon cornflour
salt, to taste
³/₄ teaspoon ground cumin
1 tablespoon lemon juice
3 tablespoons water
1 tablespoon safflower or peanut oil
¹/₄ teaspoon cumin seeds
3 tablespoons chopped fresh coriander

Steam the beans for 10 minutes. Drain, refresh under cold water and slice into thin rounds, about ¹/₂ inch thick. Set aside.

In a small bowl combine the yoghurt, green chilli, salt, cornflour, ground cumin and lemon juice. Add 3 tablespoons water and mix well.

Heat the oil in a wide, heavy-bottomed frying pan or wok over a medium–high heat. Add the cumin seeds, stir-fry for 20 seconds and add the beans. Cook, tossing, for 1 minute, then reduce the heat to low. Add the yoghurt mixture, stir everything together well, cover and simmer for 15 minutes over a low heat, stirring from time to time. Stir in the chopped fresh coriander, correct the seasonings and serve with hot cooked grains.

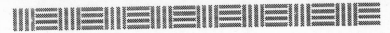

Sautéed Okra and Tomatoes

serves 4–6

1 tablespoon olive oil
1 large onion, chopped
2 cloves garlic, finely chopped or put through a press
1 hot green chilli pepper, chopped
1lb (450g) okra, trimmed just below the stem (before the seeds begin)
   and sliced 1/4–1/2 inch thick
1 tablespoon white wine vinegar
3 tablespoons white wine
1lb (450g) tomatoes, fresh or tinned, sliced
1 tablespoon chopped fresh basil or coriander
salt and freshly ground pepper, to taste

Heat the oil in a large, heavy-bottomed frying pan or casserole and add the onion and 1 clove of the garlic. Sauté over a medium heat until the onion begins to soften. Add the chilli pepper and continue to sauté for another few minutes, stirring.

Add the okra and vinegar, and sauté until the okra turns bright green: about 5 minutes. Add the wine, tomatoes and remaining garlic, and cook, stirring from time to time, for 10–15 minutes, until the okra is tender and the mixture aromatic. Add the basil or coriander and season to taste with salt and freshly ground pepper. Serve with hot cooked grains.

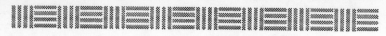

Fresh Peas with Mint and Lettuce

serves 6

3lb (1.5 kg) unshelled fresh sweet peas, shelled
5 tender lettuce leaves, cut into 1-inch *chiffonade*
1 tablespoon chopped fresh mint
salt and freshly ground pepper, to taste

Steam the peas until bright green and tender: about 10 minutes. Remove from the heat.

Wash the lettuce leaves. Heat a wide, heavy non-stick frying pan over a medium heat and add the lettuce, which should wilt in the water that remains on its leaves after washing. As soon as it wilts, add the peas and mint. Toss together, add salt and freshly ground pepper to taste, and serve at once.

Steamed Peas and Cauliflower

serves 4

1 small head cauliflower, broken into florets
1lb (450g) fresh peas, shelled; or 6oz (170g) frozen peas, thawed
salt and freshly ground pepper, to taste
fresh lemon juice (optional)
1 tablespoon chopped fresh herbs, such as parsley, basil, thyme or chervil

Steam the cauliflower for 10 minutes. Add the peas and steam for another 5–10 minutes, to taste. Toss in a serving dish with salt and freshly ground pepper to taste, the optional lemon juice and chopped fresh herbs. Serve at once.

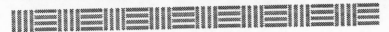

Sautéed Red and Yellow Peppers

serves 4–6

2 large sweet yellow peppers, cut in half, seeds removed, then cut
   into thin lengthwise strips
2 large sweet red peppers, cut in half, seeds removed, then cut into
   thin lengthwise strips
1 tablespoon olive oil
1–2 cloves garlic, to taste
salt and freshly ground pepper, to taste
1/4 teaspoon fresh thyme leaves (optional)

Heat the oil in a large, preferably non-stick frying pan or wok and add the
peppers and the garlic. Sauté over a medium–high heat until crisp–tender:
10–15 minutes. Add thyme and salt and pepper to taste and serve as a
side-dish.

Steamed New Potatoes with Herbs

serves 4

1 1/2lb (680g) new potatoes, scrubbed
2 teaspoons olive oil
2 tablespoons chopped fresh parsley
2 tablespoons chopped fresh dill
salt and freshly ground pepper, to taste

Cut the new potatoes in half if they are very large and place in a steamer
above boiling water. Steam for 15–20 minutes, or until tender, and
remove from the heat. Toss the potatoes with the oil, herbs and salt and
freshly ground pepper to taste, and serve.

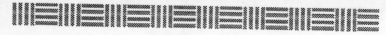

Low-fat Potato Gratin

serves 6–8

2 large cloves garlic, cut in half lengthwise
3lb (1.5kg) new potatoes, unpeeled or peeled according to your
    taste, scrubbed and sliced very thin
1½ pints (850ml) skimmed milk
2 large eggs, lightly beaten
1 teaspoon salt (or more, to taste)
a generous amount of freshly ground pepper

Pre-heat the oven to 400°F/200°C/gas mark 6. Rub the inside of a large
oval gratin dish (about 14 x 9 x 2 inches) all over with the cut side of the
garlic.

Slice the remaining garlic into thin slivers and toss with the potatoes.
Put the potatoes and garlic in an even layer in the gratin dish.

Mix together the eggs, milk and salt, and pour over the potatoes. Add
a generous amount of freshly ground pepper.

Place in the pre-heated oven and bake for about 1½–2 hours. Every
15 minutes or so, remove the casserole from the oven and, using a knife
or a wooden spoon, break up the top layer of potatoes that is drying up
and getting crusty, and fold it into the rest of the potatoes. When the
potatoes are soft, allow a golden-brown crust to form on top.

Remove from the oven and serve.

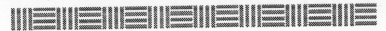

Curried Pumpkin Purée

serves 4–6

2lb (450g) fresh pumpkin
1/2 teaspoon grated fresh ginger, or 1/4 teaspoon ground ginger
1 1/2–2 teaspoons curry powder, to taste
salt and freshly ground pepper, to taste
3 tablespoons natural low-fat yoghurt

Steam the pumpkin or bake in a 400°F/200°C/gas mark 6 oven until thoroughly soft. Remove from the heat and remove the skin, stringy membranes and seeds. Purée with the remaining ingredients in a food processor, a blender or a food mill. Transfer to a lightly oiled baking dish.
    Heat through in a 350°F/180°C/gas mark 4 oven before serving.

Pumpkin and Sweet Potato Purée

serves 6–8

2lb (900g) fresh pumpkin or winter squash, seeds removed
1/2lb (225g) sweet potato, baked in its skin until tender
2–3 tablespoons freshly squeezed lime juice, to taste
3 tablespoons natural low-fat yoghurt (or more if needed)
1/4 teaspoon ground ginger
2 teaspoons curry powder (optional)
1/2 teaspoon allspice (optional)
salt and freshly ground pepper, to taste

Steam the pumpkin for 15–20 minutes, or until thoroughly tender. Drain and let drip for a few minutes in a colander. Remove the skin and stringy membranes and cut the flesh into pieces.
    Remove the skin from the baked sweet potato, and purée the potato with the pumpkin in a food processor or put through a food mill. Add the yoghurt, lime juice and spices and combine well. Add salt and freshly ground pepper to taste. Transfer to a serving dish and heat through in a medium–hot oven before serving.

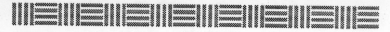

Italian-style Spinach

serves 4–6

2lb (900g) fresh spinach, or 1lb (450g) frozen spinach
1 tablespoon olive oil
1 clove garlic, finely chopped or put through a press
salt and freshly ground pepper, to taste

If using fresh spinach

Wash the spinach thoroughly and remove the stems. Heat a dry frying pan and sauté the spinach, using the liquid on the leaves as moisture, until wilted. Remove from the heat and squeeze dry.

If using frozen spinach

Let the spinach thaw, or cook it according to the instructions on the packet, and squeeze dry.

Heat the oil in a large, preferably non-stick frying pan, and sauté the garlic for about 1 minute. Add the spinach and sauté for about 2–3 minutes, stirring. Add salt and freshly ground pepper to taste and serve hot.

Baked Tomatoes

serves 4–6

4–6 firm, ripe tomatoes
2 cloves garlic, finely chopped
$1/2$ teaspoon dried thyme
$1/2$ teaspoon crumbled dried rosemary
salt and freshly ground pepper, to taste

Pre-heat the oven to 400°F/200°C/gas mark 6. Lightly oil a baking dish.

Cut a shallow cone shape out of the stem end of the tomatoes. Sprinkle the cut part with garlic, thyme, rosemary, and salt and pepper to taste.

Bake the tomatoes for about 15 minutes in the hot oven, until the skins just begin to shrivel. Serve hot.

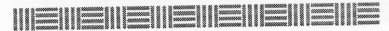

Baked Yams or Sweet Potatoes with Lime

serves 4

4 medium-sized sweet potatoes or yams
4 limes
4fl. oz (120ml) natural low-fat yoghurt (optional)

Pre-heat the oven to 425°F/220°C/gas mark 7. Scrub the potatoes and puncture the skins once with a fork. Place on a baking sheet and bake for 40–60 minutes, until thoroughly tender.

Remove the potatoes from the heat and cut them in half. Mash them with the juice of ½–1 lime for each potato, depending on your taste, and, if you wish, a tablespoon of yoghurt for each potato. Serve hot.

Spiced Vegetables en Papillote

serves 4–6

1lb (450g) new potatoes, cut into halves or quarters
2 bulbs fennel (about 1lb/450g) cut into quarters or eighths
1 head garlic, broken into cloves and peeled
4 medium-sized onions, quartered and peeled
1 tablespoon safflower or sunflower oil
salt and freshly ground pepper, to taste
1½ teaspoons cumin or garam masala (see p. 190)

Prepare an outdoor grill or pre-heat the oven to 400°F/200°C/gas mark 6.

Cut four–six double-thickness squares of aluminium foil, about 12 inches square, and brush them with oil.

Toss together the prepared vegetables with the remaining oil, salt, freshly ground pepper and garam masala. Distribute evenly among the squares of foil.

Bring the edges of the foil up around the vegetables and crimp together tightly. Place directly on the coals of the grill or in the pre-heated oven and bake for 45 minutes. Serve directly from the foil, with hot cooked grains or pasta.

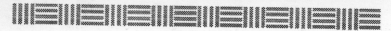

Garam Masala

makes 12 tablespoons

1½ tablespoons black or 1 tablespoon green cardamom pods
3 cinnamon sticks, each 3 inches long
1½ teaspoons whole cloves
2 tablespoons black peppercorns
4 tablespoons cumin seeds
4 tablespoons coriander seeds

Remove the seeds from the cardamom pods. Crush the cinnamon sticks with a kitchen mallet or rolling pin and combine with the other spices. Roast them in a dry frying pan or on a griddle over a medium heat, until they begin to jump around and smell toasty. Stir constantly so that they don't burn. Transfer to a bowl at once and allow to cool. Grind to a fine powder in a spice mill. Store in an air-tight container in a cool place.

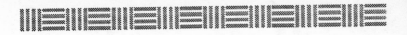

Desserts

There is no reason why you should cut out desserts on this diet. The desserts here are based on fruit, grains and low-fat yoghurt, and are only minimally sweetened. You will find here that you can make irresistible ice-creams by mashing together frozen fruit and yoghurt; they need not contain cream, eggs or sugar at all. It is easy to make a simple plate of fruit into a special dessert just by adding a little something unexpected – mint to oranges (p. 193) or lime juice to apples (p. 194). No extra sweetening is required and, naturally, the desserts which have no sugar or honey at all will contain fewer calories than the more substantial ones such as Millet Raisin Pudding (p. 205), Noodle Kugel (p. 203) or Brown Rice Pudding (p. 204). But these heavier puddings are also high in protein, and could provide you with amino acids that may be lacking in the rest of the meal. Also, leftover grain desserts could be eaten for breakfast next day.

In addition to the puddings here, remember that plain fresh fruit makes as good a dessert as anything. Buy it in season only though, or you will be disappointed.

You will see from the following recipes that this is, indeed, no diet of deprivation.

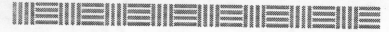

Fruit Salads

There are all kinds of combinations of fruits that you can use for fruit salads. What you choose should depend primarily on the season – i.e. what's available. Quantities for fruit salad should range from ½–1 fruit per person, or 3–6oz (85–170g) fruit per person, depending on how much fruit you eat during the rest of the day. If you have already eaten three pieces of fruit during the course of the day, then eat 3oz (85g) or ½ fruit at night.

In addition to the variety of fruits you can use for a fruit salad, there are a number of ways you can dress them up. Below are suggestions for the salads and garnishes.

blueberries and peaches or nectarines
blueberries and oranges
oranges, grapefruit and pears
apples, bananas and pears
pineapples, strawberries and oranges
assorted melon balls
cantaloupe and berries
melon, strawberry and pineapple
papaya and strawberries
mangoes and strawberries
kiwi, strawberries and oranges
fresh figs and grapes
mixed berries

Suggested Garnishes

for a fruit salad for 4–6 people

fresh chopped mint
2 tablespoons raisins or currants
2 tablespoons sunflower seeds
freshly squeezed lemon, lime or orange juice
fresh or powdered ginger
ground cinnamon or nutmeg

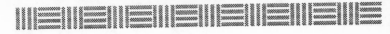

Winter Fruit Ambrosia

serves 4–6

2 oranges, peeled, white pith removed, and cut into sections
1 grapefruit, peeled, white pith removed, cut into sections
1oz (30g) chopped dates or figs
2 tablespoons chopped or slivered almonds
1 apple, cored and chopped
juice of ½ lime
1 tablespoon unsweetened grated coconut

Toss together all the ingredients. Serve at once, or refrigerate until ready
to serve.

Oranges with Figs

serves 4–6

3–4 oranges, peeled, white pith cut away, and cut into sections
2oz (55g) chopped dried figs
½ teaspoon cinnamon

Toss together the oranges, figs and cinnamon and serve, or refrigerate and
serve cold.

Oranges with Mint

serves 4–6

3–4 oranges, peeled, white pith cut away, and cut into sections
2 tablespoons chopped fresh mint (or more, to taste)

Toss together the oranges and mint. Serve at once, or refrigerate for up
to 1 hour.

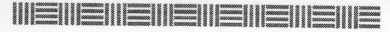

Apples with Lime Juice

serves 4–6

A very simple, refreshing dessert.

4–6 Granny Smith or Cox apples, cored and sliced
juice of 2 limes

Toss the sliced apples with the lime juice and refrigerate until ready to serve.

Yoghurt with Berries

serves 4

1lb (450g) fresh or frozen (without sugar) berries, such as blueberries,
   raspberries, blackberries or strawberries
juice of ½ lemon
1 tablespoon mild-flavoured honey (optional)
¾ pint (425ml) natural low-fat yoghurt

Using the back of a spoon, a mixer or a food processor, mash half the berries along with the lemon juice and honey. Stir together the mashed berries with the remaining berries and the yoghurt, and serve. Alternatively, place the yoghurt in individual bowls and top with the berry mixture.

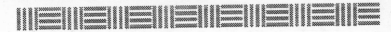

Fresh Apricot Purée

¾ pint (425ml)

This will work only with sweet, ripe apricots.

2lb (900g) sweet, fresh, ripe apricots

Bring a large pan of water to the boil. Drop in the apricots and boil for 20 seconds. Drain and run under cold water.
 Remove the skins, cut the apricots in half and remove the stones. Place in a non-corrosive saucepan (enamel, copper or stainless steel) and bring to a simmer over a medium–low heat. Simmer for 10–15 minutes, stirring every now and again, until the apricots have broken down into a thick purée. Remove from the heat and cool.
 Store in a clean, dry jar in the refrigerator. It will keep for up to a month. This makes a fabulous dessert on its own, or mixed with natural low-fat yoghurt (see below). It can also be spread on toast like jam.

Yoghurt with Apricot Purée

serves 4

¾ pint (425ml) natural low-fat yoghurt
8 heaped tablespoons Apricot Purée (see above)

Divide the yoghurt into bowls and top with the Apricot Purée.

Apple Purée

The Apple Purée on p. 25 can be served as a dessert, on its own or with natural low-fat yoghurt, or as an apple sauce.

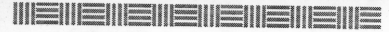

Pear Compôte

serves 6

1 pint (570ml) apple juice
2 teaspoons vanilla essence
juice of 1 lemon
1 stick cinnamon, or ½ teaspoon ground cinnamon
3 tablespoons raisins
6 firm, ripe pears
4fl. oz (120ml) natural low-fat yoghurt, for topping (optional)

Combine the apple juice, vanilla essence, lemon juice, cinnamon and
raisins in a saucepan large enough to accommodate the pears. Bring to a
simmer and simmer for 5 minutes.

Peel, core and quarter the pears and drop them immediately into the
simmering apple juice. Poach in the juice for 8–10 minutes. Remove from
the heat. Serve warm or cooled, spooning the liquid over the pears and
topping if you wish with a spoonful of natural low-fat yoghurt.

Dried Fruit Compôte with Yoghurt

serves 4–6

5oz (140g) dried apricots
5oz (140g) dried prunes
4 tablespoons raisins
2oz (55g) chopped dried pears or peaches
1 stick cinnamon
¼–½ teaspoon freshly grated nutmeg, to taste
1½ pints (850ml) water
8fl. oz (225ml) natural low-fat yoghurt

Place the dried fruit and cinnamon stick in a saucepan and cover with the
water. Bring to a simmer and simmer for 30 minutes. Serve topped with
natural low-fat yoghurt.

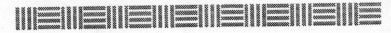

Baked Apples

serves 4

4 tart apples
4fl. oz (120ml) apple juice
cinnamon and nutmeg, to taste
2 teaspoons vanilla essence
2 tablespoons raisins
4 tablespoons natural low-fat yoghurt, for topping

Pre-heat the oven to 350°F/180°C/gas mark 4. Lightly butter a baking dish.

Cut a cone-shaped cavity into the stem end of each apple and spoon a tablespoon of apple juice into each one. Sprinkle on cinnamon and nutmeg to taste, ½ teaspoon vanilla essence per apple and the raisins. Add the remaining apple juice to the pan. Bake until tender – about 45 minutes – basting from time to time with the apple juice in the pan. Serve topped with natural low-fat yoghurt.

Baked Pears

serves 4–6

4–6 pears, peeled, cored and quartered
4fl. oz (120ml) apple juice
cinnamon and nutmeg, to taste
natural low-fat yoghurt, for topping (optional)

Pre-heat the oven to 350°F/180°C/gas mark 4.

Place the peeled, cored and quartered pears in a baking dish and pour in the apple juice. Sprinkle with cinnamon and nutmeg, and cover the dish with foil or a lid.

Bake in the pre-heated oven for 30 minutes, until the pears are soft but not mushy, and aromatic. Serve hot or cool, with a spoonful or two of the apple juice. Top, if you wish, with natural low-fat yoghurt.

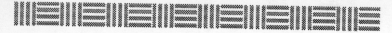

Poached Bananas

serves 4

³/4 pint (425ml) apple juice
juice of ¹/2 lemon
2 tablespoons raisins
1 teaspoon vanilla essence
a 3-inch stick of cinnamon
3 ripe but firm bananas
freshly grated nutmeg, to taste
4fl. oz (120ml) natural low-fat yoghurt

Combine the apple juice, lemon juice, raisins, vanilla essence and cinnamon in a large saucepan and bring to a simmer. Simmer for 5 minutes.
Peel the bananas and slice them into the mixture. Simmer for another 10
minutes. Sprinkle on fresh nutmeg and serve, garnishing each serving with
a dollop of yoghurt. The bananas can be served hot, warm or at room
temperature. The leftovers (if there are any) are good on hot cereal, with
additional yoghurt.

Banana–Yoghurt Ice-cream

serves 4

This is as satisfying as ice-cream, even though it has no cream or sugar in
it. You must remember to freeze the bananas in advance; it's always nice
to have them on hand anyway for snacks. You need a food processor for
this, and if you like ice-cream it's worth investing in one just for desserts
like this one.

4 medium-sized ripe bananas, peeled and frozen
8fl. oz (225ml) natural low-fat yoghurt
2–3 teaspoons vanilla essence, to taste
nutmeg, to taste

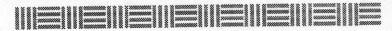

Cut the frozen bananas into chunks and place them in the food processor with the remaining ingredients. Using the start–stop action, blend together until the mixture begins to be smooth. From time to time you might have to remove pieces of banana from the blades. Make sure you use the start–stop action and not the continuous action at first, or your ice-cream will become too liquid. After about 20–25 pulses of the start–stop action, turn on the continuous action for a few seconds, until the mixture is smooth. Serve at once. (If you can't serve at once, place in the freezer. Allow to soften for 30 minutes in the refrigerator before serving.)

Strawberry or Raspberry Ice

serves 4

1 lb (450g) frozen strawberries or raspberries
1 tablespoon mild-flavoured honey
1 tablespoon lemon juice
1/2 teaspoon ground cinnamon
8fl. oz (225ml) natural low-fat yoghurt

Place all the ingredients in a food processor and pulse on and off until the berries are mashed, then purée until the mixture is smooth. Serve at once, or store in the freezer.

Note When you store this in the freezer it will freeze solid. Let it soften in the refrigerator for 30 minutes before serving. You can also make ice-lollies by freezing the mixture in moulds or paper cups, inserting a lolly stick into the middle of each one.

Vegan version

Omit the yoghurt. Add 4fl. oz (120ml) apple juice. In a food processor chop the frozen fruit with the apple juice and serve at once. This will be more like a sorbet or granita than an ice-cream.

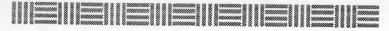

Orange Ice

serves 4–6

1 1/2 pints (850ml) orange juice from unsweetened concentrate

Place the orange juice in an ice-cream maker or sherbet-maker and process until frozen.

You can make this without an ice-cream maker by freezing the juice in ice-cube trays (without the separators) and, after 1 hour in the freezer, breaking it up in a food processor or electric mixer. Return to the freezer and freeze until just about frozen solid. Break up and freeze once more before serving. Allow to soften in the refrigerator for 20 minutes before serving.

Frozen Apple Yoghurt

serves 4

3/4 pint (425ml) natural low-fat yoghurt
10 tablespoons Apple Purée (see p. 25)
2 teaspoons mild-flavoured honey
2 teaspoons vanilla essence

Blend together all the ingredients and pour into a freezer container, or into paper cups for ice-lollies. For lollies, cover each cup with foil and insert lolly sticks into the middle of each one. (You can also use moulds.) Freeze for several hours or overnight. If you freeze this in a container and eat it like ice-cream, soften it for 30 minutes in the refrigerator before eating.

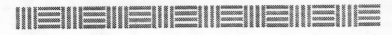

Apple Crisp

serves 6

6 tart apples, such as Granny Smith or Cox
juice of 1 lemon
1 teaspoon cinnamon
1/2 teaspoon nutmeg
1/2 teaspoon ground cloves
1 tablespoon cornflour dissolved in 2 tablespoons water
2 teaspoons vanilla essence

For the topping

6oz (170g) flaked oats
2oz (55g) wholemeal flour
1/4 teaspoon salt
2 teaspoons cinnamon
1 teaspoon allspice
2oz (55g) low-fat margarine
4 tablespoons mild-flavoured honey
6 tablespoons natural low-fat yoghurt, for topping

Pre-heat the oven to 375°F/190°C/gas mark 5. Oil or butter a 3-pint (1.5-litre) baking dish.

Combine the apples, lemon juice, cinnamon, nutmeg and cloves, the cornflour dissolved in the water, and the vanilla essence. Spread evenly in the prepared baking dish.

Using a food processor, or in a bowl with a wooden spoon, mix together the ingredients for the topping and combine well. Spread evenly over the apple mixture.

Bake for 30–45 minutes, until the top is brown and crisp. Serve warm, topped with natural low-fat yoghurt.

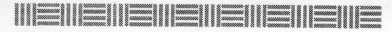

Cheesecake

serves 6–8

This can be eaten for dessert, or for a high-protein breakfast.

For the crust

2oz (55g) toasted muesli
2 tablespoons melted low-fat margarine
1 tablespoon mild-flavoured honey

For the filling

4 eggs
1lb (450g) low-fat cottage cheese
4fl. oz (120ml) natural low-fat yoghurt
2 teaspoons vanilla essence
2 tablespoons lemon juice
4 tablespoons mild-flavoured honey
1/2 teaspoon cinnamon
2 teaspoons cornflour
freshly ground nutmeg, to taste (optional)

For the topping

1 pint (570ml) natural low-fat yoghurt
1 teaspoon vanilla essence
1 tablespoon mild-flavoured honey

Pre-heat the oven to 350°F/180°C/gas mark 4. Lightly butter a 2-pint (1.2-litre) rectangular baking dish. Combine the ingredients for the crust and spread evenly in the baking dish.

Blend together the ingredients for the filling in a food processor or a blender. Pour into the baking dish and bake for 30 minutes.

Stir together the ingredients for the topping and gently spread over the top of the cheesecake. Continue to bake for another 10–15 minutes, until firm. Cool for 1 hour, then chill.

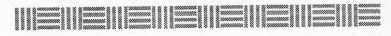

Noodle Kugel

serves 6

This recipe, from my *Fast Vegetarian Feasts*, makes a filling, high-protein dessert. You could also eat it for breakfast.

2 eggs
I egg white
8fl. oz (225ml) natural low-fat yoghurt
4oz (115g) low-fat cottage cheese
3 tablespoons mild-flavoured honey
I tablespoon grated lemon rind
¹/₂–I teaspoon cinnamon, to taste
¹/₄–¹/₂ teaspoon nutmeg, to taste
I teaspoon vanilla essence
3 tablespoons currants or raisins
I apple, chopped
4oz (115g) flat wholemeal noodles or macaroni

Pre-heat the oven to 325°F/170°C/gas mark 3 and lightly butter a 3–4-pint (2–3-litre) baking dish.

Begin heating a large pan of water for the noodles. In a large bowl, beat the eggs and egg white together with the yoghurt, cottage cheese, honey, lemon zest, cinnamon, nutmeg and vanilla essence. Stir in the raisins and apples.

Cook the pasta *al dente* – just firm to the bite – and drain. Rinse with cold water in a colander and shake out the excess water. Add to the egg mixture and combine well. Turn into the buttered casserole and cover with foil or a lid.

Bake for 35–45 minutes, until the mixture is firm and a crust has begun to form around the outside. Remove from the oven and allow to stand for 15 minutes before serving.

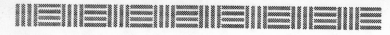

Brown Rice Pudding

serves 4–6

This is a great way to use up leftover brown rice. It makes a nourishing breakfast as well as a dessert or snack.

2 eggs
8fl. oz (225ml) skimmed milk
a pinch of salt
4 tablespoons mild-flavoured honey
I teaspoon vanilla essence
1/2 teaspoon ground cinnamon
1/4 teaspoon nutmeg
grated rind of I lemon
3 tablespoons raisins
2 small apples, peeled, cored and chopped
8oz (225g) cooked brown rice
4fl. oz (120ml) natural low-fat yoghurt or skimmed milk, for topping

Pre-heat the oven to 325°F/170°C/gas mark 3 and lightly butter a 3-pint (1.5-litre) baking dish.

Beat the eggs together with the milk, salt and honey. Stir in the vanilla essence, lemon rind, spices, raisins and apples. Fold in the cooked brown rice.

Turn the mixture into the prepared baking dish and bake for 50 minutes, or until set. Serve warm or cool, topped if you wish with natural low-fat yoghurt or warm skimmed milk.

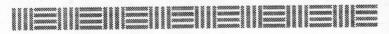

Millet Raisin Pudding

serves 4–6

A substantial dessert that also makes a good breakfast.

6oz (170g) raw millet
1½ pints (850ml) skimmed milk; or use half water, half skimmed milk
¼ teaspoon salt
2 teaspoons vanilla essence
4 tablespoons mild-flavoured honey
½ teaspoon cinnamon
½ teaspoon nutmeg
3oz (85g) raisins

Pre-heat the oven to 350°F/180°C/gas mark 4. Combine the millet and milk (or water and milk) in a saucepan and bring to the boil on top of the stove. Remove from the heat at once and stir in the remaining ingredients.

Oil a 3-pint (1.5-litre) baking dish and fill it with the millet mixture. Cover with foil or a lid and bake for 30–40 minutes, until the liquid is absorbed.

Vegan version

A vegan version of this can be made with soya milk, or by substituting all water for the milk.

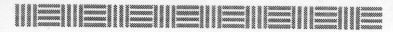

Peach Cobbler with Cornbread Topping

serves 6–8

This dessert tastes like a big splurge, yet it hardly has any sugar at all.

For the filling

2lb (900g) ripe peaches, sliced
2 teaspoons vanilla essence
1/2 teaspoon cinnamon
juice of 1/2 lemon
1 tablespoon cornflour or arrowroot

For the topping

2oz (55g) wholemeal pastry flour
6oz (170g) stoneground yellow cornmeal
1 tablespoon baking powder
1/4 teaspoon salt
2 eggs
8fl. oz (225ml) skimmed milk or natural low-fat yoghurt
4 tablespoons mild-flavoured honey
2 tablespoons safflower or sunflower oil

For garnish

natural low-fat yoghurt, 1 tablespoon per serving

Pre-heat the oven to 350°F/180°C/gas mark 4. Grease a 9 x 13-inch baking dish or a 10–12-inch pie plate with margarine.

Toss together the peaches, vanilla and cinnamon. Dissolve the cornflour or arrowroot in the lemon juice and mix with the peaches.

Sift together the flour, cornmeal, baking powder and salt. In a separate bowl beat together the eggs, milk or yoghurt, honey and oil. Fold into the dry ingredients and stir together thoroughly. Do not over-beat; a few lumps are OK.

Spread the peaches in the prepared baking dish. Pour the cornbread topping evenly over the peaches. It will be very runny but it will stay on the surface.

Bake the cobbler for 30–40 minutes, until the top is golden-brown and

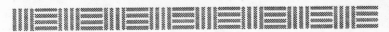

the peaches are bubbling. Remove from the oven, allow to cool for a few minutes and serve. This is good topped with natural low-fat yoghurt. It is also good cold or reheated for breakfast.

Oatmeal Raisin Biscuits

4 dozen biscuits

4fl. oz (120ml) mild-flavoured honey
4fl. oz (120ml) safflower or sunflower oil
1 egg
2 teaspoons vanilla essence
3/4 teaspoon cinnamon
1/2 teaspoon nutmeg
1/4 teaspoon ground cloves
1/4 teaspoon salt
1/2 teaspoon bicarbonate of soda
10oz (285g) flaked oats
4oz (115g) wholemeal or wholemeal pastry flour
4oz (115g) raisins

Pre-heat the oven to 350°F/180°C/gas mark 4. Oil baking sheets.

Cream together the honey and oil and beat in the egg and vanilla essence. Stir in the spices.

Mix together the salt, bicarbonate of soda, oats and flour. Stir into the wet ingredients and combine well. (This can be done in a food processor or electric mixer.) Stir in the raisins.

Drop the mixture a tablespoon at a time on to the baking sheets and bake for 12–15 minutes, until the biscuits are beginning to brown. Cool on racks.

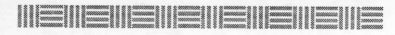

Healthy (or Healthier) Snacks for Children and Teenagers

Children and teenagers who are overweight are usually so because they eat between meals, and they eat junk food. Obesity among children is becoming a widespread problem because not enough attention is paid to the kinds of foods they eat, both at meals and between meals. Sugar and fats, as usual, are the culprits. They come in the form of sweets and fried foods.

Snacking is a phenomenon that isn't going to go away, so the only solution is to reduce the potential damage by creating alternative snacks. The recipes below don't pretend to taste exactly like junk foods; but they will satisfy the same cravings for foods like chocolate, ice-cream and crisps – cravings for sugar and salt. Nor do I claim that these are all low in calories, but they're much less fattening than their equivalents.

Chocolate

Carob makes a wonderful substitute for chocolate. It is a powder ground from the pods of the St John's bean tree, and has a chocolatey flavour with only half the fat, lots of minerals and natural sugar.

Carob Syrup
2 tablespoons low-fat margarine
2 tablespoons carob powder
1 tablespoon low-fat milk powder
4 tablespoons demerara sugar
1/2 teaspoon vanilla essence
skimmed milk, as needed

Beat together the margarine, carob powder and milk powder in a saucepan. Add the sugar and melt together over a low heat. Stir in the vanilla. Thin out to the desired consistency with skimmed milk.

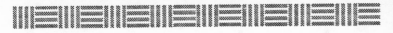

Hot Carob Chocolate

2 servings

³/₄ pint (425ml) skimmed milk
4 tablespoons carob powder
1 tablespoon mild-flavoured honey

Blend together all the ingredients and heat to a simmer over a medium heat.

Carob Fudge

16 pieces

4 tablespoons demerara sugar
4 tablespoons carob powder
6 tablespoons low-fat milk powder
4fl. oz (120ml) water
a pinch salt
1 tablespoon low-fat margarine
¹/₂ teaspoon vanilla essence
4 tablespoons walnuts or sunflower seeds (optional)

Combine the sugar, carob powder, milk powder, water and salt in a saucepan and bring to a simmer over a low heat. Stir to melt the sugar, then simmer for 10–15 minutes without stirring, until the mixture is thick.

Remove from the heat and add the margarine and the vanilla essence. Beat for 5 minutes in an electric mixer. Stir in the optional walnuts or sunflower seeds. Spread out the mixture in an oiled tin and refrigerate until solid. Cut into squares. Keep refrigerated.

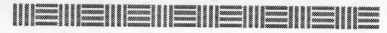

Carob Brownies

12 brownies

4fl. oz (120ml) sunflower or safflower oil
3fl. oz (90ml) mild-flavoured honey
2 tablespoons black treacle
2 eggs, beaten
1 teaspoon vanilla essence
3oz (85g) wholemeal pastry flour
1 teaspoon double-acting baking powder
1/4 teaspoon salt
2oz (55g) carob powder
2oz (55g) sunflower seeds

Pre-heat the oven to 350°F/180°C/gas mark 4 and oil a 9-inch-square baking tin.

Cream together the oil, honey and treacle, then beat in the eggs and vanilla essence. Sift together the flour, baking powder and salt. Stir into the liquid mixture, then stir in the carob and sunflower seeds. Mix well.

Spread the batter in the oiled tin and bake for 30–40 minutes, until a tester comes out clean. Allow to cool in the tin, then cut into squares. Wrap in plastic or foil.

These are more crumbly than chocolate brownies.

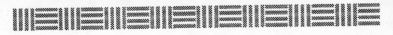

Sodas

Wholefood shops now stock numerous brands of sodas made without sugar, colourings or additives. There are also sparkling fruit juices, which easily satisfy the need for something bubbly and sweet.

Better still – and cheaper – you can make your own, using one part fruit juice and one part soda water or sparkling mineral water.

Fruit Soda 1

2 servings

$^1/_2$ pint (285ml) any fruit juice
$^1/_2$ pint (285ml) soda water or sparkling mineral water

Fruit Soda 2

3 servings

$^1/_2$ pint (285ml) orange juice
$^1/_2$ pint (285ml) soda water or sparkling mineral water
$^1/_2$ pint (285ml) cranberry juice

Fruit Soda 3

4 servings

1 small tin frozen fruit-juice concentrate
2 pints (1.2 litres) soda water or sparkling mineral water

Dissolve the fruit-juice concentrate in the soda water or sparkling mineral water and serve, or refrigerate in a sealed bottle.

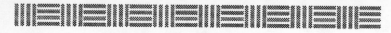

Crisps and Savoury Snacks

Homemade Low-fat Potato Crisps

serves 1

1 potato, unpeeled and sliced very thin

Pre-heat the oven to 325°F/170°C/gas mark 3. Place the potato slices on a non-stick baking sheet. Bake for 40 minutes, or until thoroughly crisp and brown.

Banana Crisps

Pre-heat the oven to 225°F/110°C/gas mark ¼. Slice bananas thin and toss them with the juice of 1 lemon. Place on non-stick baking sheets and bake for 2–3 hours, until thoroughly crisp and golden.

Aubergine Crisps

Slice a long, thin aubergine into thin slices. Salt the slices and weight them down with a board for 1 hour to draw out the bitterness. Rinse and pat dry.

Meanwhile, pre-heat the oven to 250°F/130°C/gas mark ½. Place the aubergine slices on non-stick baking sheets and bake for 1 hour, or until thoroughly crisp.

Courgette Crisps

Pre-heat the oven to 250°F/130°C/gas mark ½. Slice the courgettes thin and bake on non-stick baking sheets for 1 hour, or until thoroughly crisp.

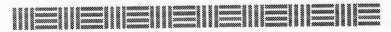

Homemade Low-fat Tortilla Crisps

12 corn tortillas, cut into wedges

Pre-heat the oven to 250°F/130°C/gas mark ½. Place the tortilla wedges on non-stick baking sheets and bake for 40 minutes, or until crisp and beginning to brown.

Popcorn

Pop your own in a dry electric popcorn popper, or using a small amount of sunflower oil. Instead of tossing with butter and salt, try other seasonings, like curry powder, dry mustard, paprika, kelp, cumin. Popcorn is one of the easiest low-calorie snacks.

Ice-cream

Both supermarkets and wholefood shops now stock fruit ices made from fruit juice, with no extra sugar, and you can find ice-cream made with honey instead of sugar in wholefood shops. Frozen yoghurt and ice-milk sweetened with honey are better nutritional buys than regular ice-cream.

See recipes for Banana–Yoghurt Ice-cream, Strawberry or Raspberry Ice, Frozen Apple Yoghurt (pp. 198, 199 and 200).

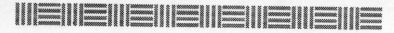

Frozen Fruit Bites

Freeze bite-sized fruit, like grapes, strawberries, berries and banana slices tossed in lemon juice. These make fabulous, low-calorie frozen treats.

Seedless grapes or berries

Remove grapes from stems, freeze grapes and berries in plastic bags.

Bananas

Slice and toss with lemon juice. Lay the slices on pieces of greaseproof paper, cover with another sheet of greaseproof paper and freeze in a plastic bag.

Frozen banana sticks

Peel bananas and cut them in half crosswise. Toss with lemon juice. Insert lolly sticks and freeze in plastic bags.

Frozen carob-coated banana sticks

Peel bananas, cut them in half crosswise, toss with lemon juice and freeze as above. When frozen, dip in carob syrup (see p. 208) and return to the freezer.

Fruit-juice Ice-lollies

Freeze fruit juice in moulds (available at supermarkets and kitchen-supply stores), or in paper cups. Cover the cups with foil and insert sticks in the middle. The foil holds up the stick.

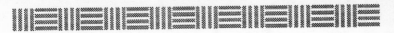

Frozen Yoghurt Lollies

Blend together natural low-fat yoghurt and fresh fruit, such as berries or bananas, or try yoghurt and fruit-juice concentrate. Freeze in moulds or paper cups, as above. Try the following combinations:

Mixed Fruit and Yoghurt Lollies

serves 6

1 pear, chopped
10oz (285g) strawberries, frozen or fresh
4fl. oz (120ml) natural low-fat yoghurt
1/2 banana

Blend together all the ingredients until smooth, and freeze in moulds or paper cups.

Banana–Orange–Yoghurt Lollies

serves 6

8fl. oz (225ml) natural yoghurt (or buttermilk)
4fl. oz (120ml) orange juice, fresh or from concentrate
1 banana

Blend together all the ingredients until smooth, and freeze in moulds or paper cups.

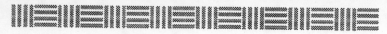

Strawberry–Yoghurt Lollies

serves 6

8fl. oz (225ml) natural low-fat yoghurt (or buttermilk)
a 10oz (285g) packet frozen strawberries
1 tablespoon mild-flavoured honey

Blend together all the ingredients until smooth, and freeze in ice-lolly moulds or paper cups.

Pineapple–Banana–Mint Lollies

serves 6

³/₄ pint (425ml) pineapple juice
1 banana
1 tablespoon fresh mint

Blend together all the ingredients until smooth, and freeze in ice-lolly moulds or paper cups.

Yoghurt Cream Lollies

serves 6

³/₄ pint (425ml) natural low-fat yoghurt
1 tablespoon vanilla essence
1 tablespoon mild-flavoured honey
8fl. oz (225ml) orange juice from concentrate

Blend together all the ingredients until smooth, and freeze in ice-lolly moulds or paper cups.

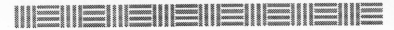

Carob Fudge Lollies

serves 6

8fl. oz (225ml) skimmed milk
8fl. oz (225ml) natural low-fat yoghurt
3 tablespoons carob powder
2 tablespoons mild-flavoured honey
1 teaspoon vanilla essence

Blend together all the ingredients until smooth, and freeze in ice-lolly moulds or paper cups.

Pizza

If snacking on fast-food pizza, remove the cheese and sausage, and ask them not to douse the pizza with oil.

Many wholefood shops sell pizza with wholemeal crusts. If they don't have assembled pizzas, they almost all now stock frozen wholemeal crusts, as well as several varieties of bottled tomato sauce. Armed with these ingredients you can put together your own pizzas in no time. If you can't find any of these things, try the recipes on pp. 152–5.

A desire for pizza may be nothing more than a desire for that wonderful taste of bread and Italian tomato sauce. This craving can be satisfied with wholemeal English muffins, pitta or bread, spread with tomato sauce, sprinkled with a little low-fat Mozzarella or dry, crumbly white cheese and toasted under the grill or in the oven. In fact, pizza can be one of the healthier snacks, as long as you follow these recommendations.

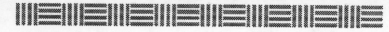

Fruit

Certainly fruit is one of the best items for snacking. Try to vary your selection. If you are watching your calories, stick to no more than three pieces a day.

Carrots and Other Vegetables

Eat as many carrots as you want. Try these other vegetables too. They are the best snacks of all, because you can eat as much as you feel like:

asparagus
green beans
beetroot
broccoli
cabbage
cauliflower
celery

courgettes
cucumbers
lettuce of all kinds
mushrooms
red or green peppers
tomatoes

Season them with the following dips:

plain mustard
vinegar
lemon juice
soy sauce
any of the low-fat dressings on pp. 53–4
Salsa Fresca (p. 55)
low-fat yoghurt with added herbs or spices
cottage cheese with chives
any of the low-fat spreads on pp. 46–8

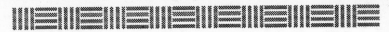

Toast

Use wholemeal breads and replace butter with low-fat, additive-free margarine, unsweetened fruit preserves or fruit purées (see pp. 25 and 195), or *fromage blanc*.

Biscuits and Pastries

If pastries are a weakness, try the muffins or the oatmeal biscuits on pp. 26–33 and 207.

The recipes below are for wholesome (though not low-calorie) biscuits for children.

Peanut Butter–Banana Biscuits

4 dozen biscuits

4 tablespoons sunflower or safflower oil
6 tablespoons mild-flavoured honey
2 eggs
1/2 teaspoon vanilla essence
8 tablespoons natural peanut butter
1 large ripe banana, mashed
3oz (85g) wholemeal pastry flour
2 teaspoons double-acting baking powder
1/4 teaspoon salt

Pre-heat the oven to 350°F/180°C/gas mark 4. Lightly oil non-stick baking sheets.

Cream together the oil and honey. Beat in the eggs, vanilla essence, peanut butter and mashed banana. Sift together the flour, baking powder and salt and stir into the liquid mixture. Blend well.

Drop the mixture on to prepared baking sheets in scant tablespoonfuls and bake for 12–15 minutes. Cool on racks.

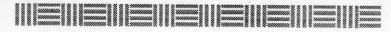

Carob-chip Biscuits

4 dozen

4fl. oz (120ml) sunflower or safflower oil
6 tablespoons mild-flavoured honey
2 eggs
1 teaspoon vanilla essence
8oz (225g) sifted wholemeal pastry flour
1 teaspoon baking powder
¼ teaspoon salt
5oz (140g) carob chips

Pre-heat the oven to 375°F/190°C/gas mark 5. Lightly oil non-stick baking sheets.

Cream together the oil and honey. Beat in the eggs and vanilla essence. Sift together flour, baking powder and salt and stir into the wet ingredients. Stir in the carob chips.

Drop in heaped teaspoonfuls on to the baking sheets and bake for 12 minutes. Cool on racks.

Diet plans for children

You never know what children are and are not going to like. I would use the first or second diet plan and, if you find that your children like only certain dishes, concentrate on those. They are all healthy and designed with protein balance and maximum nutrition in mind, so it won't make much difference nutritionally if you repeat the same meals often during the week.

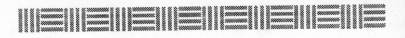

THE MENU PLANS

Introducing the Menu Plans

Here are a number of menu plans to choose from. If you are making a transition to vegetarianism, begin with the first one, which contains a few meat and fish dishes. The second plan is totally vegetarian, and the third one is for vegans – those of you who include no dairy products or eggs in your diet.

With the exception of the Quick Weight-loss Plan, these are menu plans for gradual weight loss. The meals are filling and satisfying, but the overall calorie and fat content is low.

What to drink

Alcoholic beverages are high in empty calories: 12fl. oz beer or ale contain 140–150 calories; wine contains 87 calories per 3½fl. oz (100ml) serving, and distilled spirits contain 97–124 calories per 1½fl. oz (45ml) serving. So, obviously, it will be easier for you to lose weight if you limit your alcohol consumption.

This said, the diets are sufficiently low in calories to allow for a glass of wine from time to time. Without making any strict rules, I would recommend no more than a glass of wine per day. Less is better. Water is best. Iced herbal teas, especially mint teas, make very nice accompaniments to meals. Make up a jug in the morning and have it on hand in the fridge to drink with lunch and dinner.

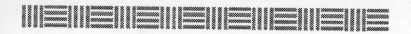

A Gradual Weight–loss Plan

Here are three weeks of menus, with a mix of vegetarian meals and menus containing fish, chicken or rabbit. The fat and, hence, calories in the chicken have been very much reduced by removing the skin. Naturally, these are only suggestions; there are plenty of other recipes in this book to choose from .

This is not a crash diet. It's a gradual one, based on my firm belief that crash dieting doesn't work. For one thing, when you starve yourself, your body thinks there is a famine, and slows down its metabolism so that you burn calories more slowly. That's exactly what you don't want. Rather, this is a lifestyle diet. The bulk of the calories are complex carbohydrates, the quickest burning type. There are very little fat calories, and your body will soon begin to burn up the excess fat it has been carrying.

You won't go hungry with these menus. But you needn't feel bound to them. If you like one kind of breakfast every day, by all means eat it every day. And if your stomach doesn't wake up until lunch because you dine late at night, don't feel you have to eat breakfast. If you like a certain dish and could eat it more than once a week, do so. Also, there are many delicious recipes which don't show up here, so make sure you've had a healthy browse through the recipes before you settle on this particular sequence.

If you find that you want to lose weight more quickly, reduce portions, eliminate desserts and/or bread, and see the menu plan on page 243.

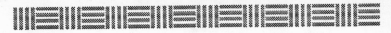

Week 1

Monday

Breakfast
6fl. oz (180ml) natural low-fat
    yoghurt with 1 tablespoon
    Apricot Purée
1 muffin or 1 slice wholemeal toast
    spread with Apricot Purée
4fl. oz (120ml) orange juice

Lunch
Lentil Salad
Wholemeal bread
1 piece fruit

Dinner
Chicken and Vegetable Curry
Bulgur
Carrot–Apple Salad
Banana–Yoghurt Ice-cream

Tuesday

Breakfast
½ grapefruit
1 soft-boiled egg
Wholemeal toast with Apricot
    Purée

Lunch
Tabouli (use last night's bulgur)
Crudités
1 piece fruit

Dinner
Red Cabbage and Apple Soup
Wholemeal bread
Tossed Mixed Green Salad
Yoghurt with Berries

Wednesday

Breakfast
Banana–Yoghurt Smoothie
1 Bran Muffin (or other muffin of
    your choice – see pp. 26–33)

Lunch
Tofu Salad Sandwich
1 piece fruit

Dinner
Steamed Cod Fillets with
    Tomato–Caper Sauce
Wholemeal bread
Tossed Mixed Green Salad with
    Low-fat Dressing
Orange Ice

Thursday

Breakfast
Fruity Oatmeal
4fl. oz (120ml) orange or grape-
    fruit juice

Lunch
Tuna Salad Pitta
Crudités
1 piece fruit

Dinner
Crustless Tofu Quiche
Steamed Greens with Vinegar or
    Lemon Juice
Watercress and Mushroom Salad,
    or Tossed Mixed Green Salad
Strawberry Ice

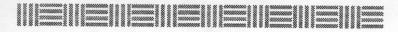

Friday

Breakfast
Unsweetened muesli with milk
   and/or apple juice
1 banana
4fl. oz (120ml) orange or grapefruit juice

Lunch
Curried Brown Rice Salad
4fl. oz (120ml) natural low-fat
   yoghurt with 1 tablespoon
   Apricot Purée

Dinner
Fish Teriyaki
Brown rice
Steamed broccoli
Baked Apple

Saturday

Breakfast
Oatmeal Pancakes
Apple Purée
4fl. oz (120ml) orange juice

Lunch
Corn Chowder
Wholemeal bread
Tomato Salad
1 piece fruit

Dinner
Grilled Chicken Breasts
Steamed Artichokes with Tofu
   Vinaigrette
Grated Carrot Salad, or Tossed
   Mixed Green Salad
Fruit Salad

Sunday

Breakfast
Grapefruit or melon
Mushroom Omelette
Wholemeal toast
4fl. oz (120ml) orange juice

Lunch
Oriental Beansprout Salad
Wholemeal bread
1 piece fruit

Dinner
Curried Cauliflower Soup
Tossed Mixed Green Salad
Wholemeal bread
Noodle Kugel

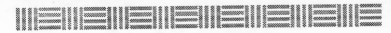

Week 2

Monday

Breakfast
1 muffin of your choice (see pp. 26–33)
4fl. oz (120ml) low-fat cottage cheese or natural low-fat yoghurt
4fl. oz (120ml) orange juice

Lunch
Egg salad sandwich
1 piece fruit

Dinner
Pasta with Creamy Tomato Sauce
Tossed Mixed Green Salad
Orange Ice

Tuesday

Breakfast
Wholemeal Buttermilk Waffles with Apple Purée or Prune Butter and natural low-fat yoghurt
4fl. oz (120ml) orange juice

Lunch
Vegetable Salad Pitta Pocket
1 piece fruit

Dinner
Black Beans
Cornbread or corn tortillas
Spinach Salad
Oranges with Mint

Wednesday

Breakfast
Scrambled Eggs
Wholemeal toast
½ grapefruit
4fl. oz (120ml) orange juice

Lunch
Black-bean Burritos with lettuce and tomatoes
1 piece fruit

Dinner
Rabbit Cooked in Chicken Stock and Wine with Fresh Peas
Tossed Mixed Green Salad
Wholemeal bread
Pear Compôte

Thursday

Breakfast
Buckwheat Pancakes with Apricot Purée and natural low-fat yoghurt
4fl. oz (120ml) orange juice

Lunch
Cucumber–Cottage Cheese Sandwich
Crudités
1 piece fruit

Dinner
Stir-fried Tofu and Vegetables
Bulgur Pilaf (make extra for tomorrow's lunch)
Oriental Beansprout Salad
Frozen Apple Yoghurt

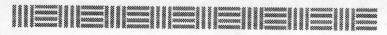

Friday

Breakfast
Hot Mixed-grains Porridge with
    Fruit
4fl. oz (120ml) skimmed milk
6fl. oz (180ml) fruit juice

Lunch
Bulgur Pilaf Salad
Crudités
1 piece fruit

Dinner
Grilled Salmon Steaks
Baked Potatoes with Low-fat
    Toppings
Baked Tomatoes
Broccoli Salad
Baked Pears

Saturday

Breakfast
Apple Smoothie
1 Orange–Apricot Muffin

Lunch
Humous
Wholemeal bread or pitta
Middle Eastern Salad

Dinner
Pizza
Tossed Mixed Green Salad
Banana–Yoghurt Ice-cream

Sunday

Breakfast
Wholemeal Bagels
Low-fat Cream Cheese
½ grapefruit or 4fl. oz (120ml)
    orange juice

Lunch
Mushroom Toasts
Italian-style Spinach
Mixed Bean Salad
1 piece fruit

Dinner
Minestrone
Wholemeal bread
Watercress and Mushroom Salad
Apples with Lime Juice

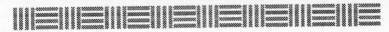

Week 3

Monday

Breakfast
Mixed-grains Porridge with
    skimmed milk
1 banana
4fl. oz (120ml) orange juice

Lunch
Gazpacho
Wholemeal bread
2oz (55g) low-fat cottage cheese
    (optional)
1 piece fruit

Dinner
Spinach Lasagne
Spinach and Tangerine Salad
Dried Fruit Compôte with Yoghurt

Tuesday

Breakfast
Scrambled Eggs
1–2 slices wholemeal toast
½ grapefruit
4fl. oz (120ml) orange juice

Lunch
Tofu and Beansprout Salad sand-
    wich or pitta pocket
Crudités
2 Oatmeal Biscuits
1 piece fruit

Dinner
Haricot Bean Soup with
    Wholemeal Croûtons
Batavia and Orange Salad, or
    Tossed Mixed Green Salad
Brown Rice Pudding, or Millet
    Pudding (make extra for
    tomorrow's breakfast)

Wednesday

Breakfast
Brown Rice Pudding, or Millet
    Pudding
4fl. oz (120ml) orange juice

Lunch
Cottage cheese and cucumber
    sandwich
Crudités
1 piece fruit

Dinner
Fish au Gros Sel
Roasted Red Peppers
Brown rice
Poached Bananas

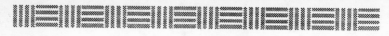

Thursday

Breakfast
Banana Smoothie
Bran Muffin or wholemal toast
    with Apple Purée

Lunch
Chinese Chicken Salad
Crudités
Wholemeal bread
1 piece fruit

Dinner
Purée of Spinach Soup
Warm Potato Salad
Wholemeal bread
Oranges with Mint

Friday

Breakfast
Couscous with Fruit
4fl. oz (120ml) orange juice

Lunch
Warm Chick-pea Salad
Wholemeal bread or pitta
1 piece fruit

Dinner
North Indian Rice Pilaf
Cucumbers Simmered in White
    Wine
Tossed Mixed Green Salad
Peach Cobbler

Saturday

Breakfast
Apple Omelette
Wholemeal toast
½ grapefruit
4fl. oz (120ml) orange juice

Lunch
Salade Niçoise
Wholemeal bread
Frozen Apple Yoghurt

Dinner
Soft Potato–Bean Tacos
Salsa Fresca
Steamed Courgettes
Mexican Corn Salad
Winter Fruit Ambrosia

Sunday

Breakfast
Cottage Cheese–Apple Pancakes
Apple Purée
4fl. oz (120ml) orange juice

Lunch
Grilled Sole or Chicken Breasts
    Baked in Foil
Wholemeal bread
Tossed Mixed Green Salad
1 piece fruit

Dinner
Cabbage Soup Chinoise
Wholemeal bread
Grated Carrot Salad
Apple Crisp

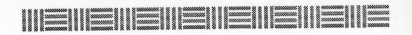

A Gradual Weight-loss Plan
for Vegetarians

This diet plan is much like the preceding one, except there is no meat. It's a sensible, high-carbohydrate diet that won't leave you hungry. Feel free to repeat menus you like, or to substitute other recipes from the book.

If you find that you want to lose weight more quickly, reduce portions, eliminate desserts and/or bread, and see the menu plan on page 243.

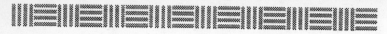

Week 1

Monday

Breakfast
Mixed-grains Porridge with Fruit
4fl. oz (120ml) orange juice

Lunch
Low-fat Egg Salad
Wholemeal bread
1 piece fruit

Dinner
Mushroom Risotto
Italian-style Spinach
Tossed Mixed Green Salad
Raspberry Ice

Tuesday

Breakfast
2 pieces wholemeal bread spread
    with 2 tablespoons Low-fat
    Cream Cheese or low-fat
    cottage cheese
1 banana
4fl. oz (120ml) orange juice

Lunch
Lentil Salad
Sliced tomatoes

Dinner
Meatless Chilli
Cornbread
Spinach Salad
Winter Fruit Ambrosia

Wednesday

Breakfast
Unsweetened muesli with
    skimmed milk and/or apple
    juice
4fl. oz (120ml) orange juice

Lunch
'Chilidogs'
Tossed Mixed Green Salad
1 piece fruit

Dinner
Corn Chowder
Wholemeal bread
Broccoli Salad
Apple Sauce with natural low-
    fat yoghurt

Thursday

Breakfast
Scrambled Eggs
Wholemeal toast
4fl. oz (120ml) orange juice

Lunch
Blender Gazpacho
Wholemeal bread
Fruit Salad

Dinner
Aubergine Moussaka
Middle Eastern Salad
Orange Ice

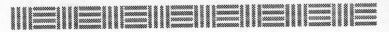

Friday

Breakfast
Fruity Oatmeal
4fl. oz (120ml) orange juice

Lunch
Tofu Salad Sandwich
Crudités
1 piece fruit

Dinner
Piperade
Steamed New Potatoes with
   Herbs
Tossed Mixed Green Salad
Apple Crisp

Saturday

Breakfast
Buckwheat Pancakes with Apple
   Purée, natural low-fat yoghurt
   or Apricot Purée
4fl. oz (120ml) orange juice or ½
   grapefruit

Lunch
Warm Chick-pea Salad
Wholemeal bread
1 piece fruit, or Oranges with Figs

Dinner
Pasta with Uncooked Tomatoes
Tossed Mixed Green Salad
Peach Cobbler

Sunday

Breakfast
Apple Omelette
Wholemeal toast with *fromage
   blanc*
4fl. oz (120ml) orange juice or ½
   grapefruit

Lunch
Puréed Pumpkin Soup
Tossed Mixed Green Salad
Fruit Salad

Dinner
Grilled Tofu 'Cutlets'
Courgettes Provençale
Cooked grains of your choice
Watercress and Mushroom Salad
Apples with Lime Juice

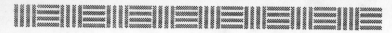

Week 2

Monday

Breakfast
Unsweetened muesli with
    skimmed milk and/or apple juice
4fl. oz (120ml) orange juice

Lunch
Chilled Yoghurt–Cucumber Soup
Wholemeal bread
1 piece fruit

Dinner
Stir-fried Tofu and Vegetables
Brown rice or millet
Oriental Beansprout Salad
Apple Purée

Tuesday

Breakfast
Banana Smoothie
Bran Muffin or 1 slice wholemeal
    toast with *fromage blanc*

Lunch
Cottage Cheese and Fruit Salad
Wholemeal bread

Dinner
Curried Brown Rice Salad
Aubergine Purée on wholemeal
    bread
Strawberry Ice

Wednesday

Breakfast
Mixed-grains Porridge with Fruit
4fl. oz (120ml) orange juice

Lunch
Pizza Sandwich
Tossed Mixed Green Salad
1 piece fruit

Dinner
Potato–Leek Soup
Broccoli Timbale
Baked Tomatoes
Fruit Salad

Thursday

Breakfast
1 soft-boiled egg
2 slices wholemeal toast
4fl. oz (120ml) orange juice or
    ½ grapefruit

Lunch
Low-fat cottage cheese
Watercress and Mushroom Salad
Wholemeal bread
1 piece fruit

Dinner
Crustless Tofu Quiche
Spiced Vegetables en Papillote
Spinach Salad
Frozen Apple Yoghurt

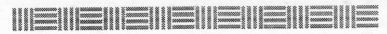

Friday

Breakfast
Unsweetened muesli with
   skimmed milk and/or apple juice
4fl. oz (120ml) orange juice

Lunch
Spinach and Tofu Pitta Sandwiches
1 piece fruit

Dinner
Hot and Sour Soup
Spicy Aubergines and Mangetouts
   with Miso
Cooked bulgur or millet
Cheesecake

Saturday

Breakfast
Cottage Cheese–Apple Pancakes
   with Apple Purée
4fl. oz (120ml) orange juice

Lunch
Tabouli
Tomato Salad
1 piece fruit

Dinner
Grated Carrot Salad
Vegetable Couscous
Oranges with Figs

Sunday

Breakfast
Wholemeal Bagels with Low-fat
   Cream Cheese and Apple
   Purée
Fruit Salad

Lunch
Apple Omelette
Tossed Mixed Green Salad

Dinner
Beetroot and Vegetable Borscht
Marinated Vegetables
Noodle Kugel

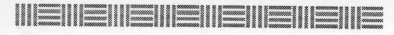

Week 3

Monday

Breakfast
6fl. oz (180ml) natural low-fat
   yoghurt with 1 tablespoon
   Apricot Purée
1 muffin (see pp. 26–33) or
   1 slice wholemeal toast spread
   with Apricot Purée
4fl. oz (120ml) orange juice

Lunch
Marinated Vegetable pittas
1 piece fruit

Dinner
Spicy Chick-pea Soup
Tossed Mixed Green Salad
Brown Rice Pudding

Tuesday

Breakfast
Brown Rice Pudding
4fl. oz (120ml) orange juice

Lunch
Low-fat Egg Salad sandwich
1 piece fruit

Dinner
Pizza
Grilled Mushrooms
Spinach Salad
Banana–Yoghurt Ice-cream

Wednesday

Breakfast
1 soft-boiled egg
2 slices wholemeal toast
4fl. oz (120ml) orange juice or
   ½ grapefruit

Lunch
Warm Potato Salad
Sliced tomatoes
1 piece fruit

Dinner
Curried Tofu and Vegetables
Saffron Millet
Tossed Mixed Green Salad
Apple Purée

Thursday

Breakfast
Fruity Oatmeal
4fl. oz (120ml) orange juice

Lunch
Cottage Cheese and Fruit Salad
Wholemeal bread

Dinner
Hearty Mushroom and Barley
   Soup
Wholemeal bread
Broccoli Salad
Baked Pears

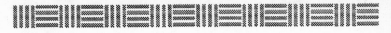

Friday

Breakfast
2 pieces wholemeal bread spread
    with 2 tablespoons Low-fat
    Cream Cheese or low-fat
    cottage cheese
1 banana
4fl. oz (120ml) orange juice

Lunch
Courgette Soup with Dill
Tossed Mixed Green Salad
Wholemeal bread
1 piece fruit

Dinner
Pasta with Broccoli and Tomato
    Sauce
Spinach and Tangerine Salad
Yoghurt with Berries or Apricot
    Purée

Saturday

Breakfast
Wholemeal Waffles with natural
    low-fat yoghurt and Apricot
    Purée
4fl. oz (120ml) orange juice

Lunch
Tofu Salad Sandwich
Crudités
1 piece fruit

Dinner
Provençal Garlic Soup
Baked Potatoes with Low-fat
    Toppings
Tossed Mixed Green Salad or
    Spinach Salad
Dried Fruit Compôte

Sunday

Breakfast
Scrambled Eggs
2 slices wholemeal toast with
    fromage blanc

Lunch
Millet–Lentil Salad
Sliced tomatoes
Apple Purée

Dinner
Minestrone
Tossed Mixed Green Salad
Wholemeal bread
Orange juice

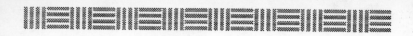

A Gradual Weight-loss Plan
for Vegans

Although vegan diets are more restricted than ovolacto vegetarian diets, there is still plenty to choose from. I have devised low-fat salad dressings that contain no yoghurt so that all the salads are viable. Again, these are just suggestions. There are plenty of other recipes to choose from. Like the preceding menu plan, this is for gradual weight-loss. It is not a crash diet; the weight you lose should stay off.

Week 1

Monday

Breakfast
Mixed-grains Porridge with Fruit
4fl. oz (120ml) orange juice

Lunch
Lentil Salad
Wholemeal bread
1 piece fruit

Dinner
Mushroom Risotto (omit
 Parmesan)
Italian-style Spinach
Tossed Mixed Green Salad
Raspberry Ice

Tuesday

Breakfast
2 pieces wholemeal bread with
 Apricot or Apple Purée
1 banana
4fl. oz (120ml) orange juice

Lunch
Curried Brown Rice Salad
Sliced tomatoes

Dinner
Meatless Chilli
Corn or wheat tortillas
Spinach Salad
Winter Fruit Ambrosia

Wednesday

Breakfast
Unsweetened muesli with apple
 juice
4fl. oz (120ml) orange juice

Lunch
'Chilidogs'
Tossed Mixed Green Salad
1 piece fruit

Dinner
Bean and Vegetable Soup
Wholemeal bread
Broccoli Salad
Apple Purée

Thursday

Breakfast
Couscous with Fruit
Wholemeal toast
4fl. oz (120ml) orange juice

Lunch
Blender Gazpacho
Wholemeal bread
Fruit Salad

Dinner
Chilled Tofu with Dipping Sauces
Marinated Vegetables
Orange Ice

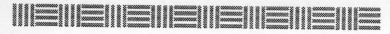

Friday

Breakfast
Fruity Oatmeal
4fl. oz (120ml) orange juice

Lunch
Tofu Salad Sandwich
Crudités
1 piece fruit

Dinner
Spicy Aubergines and Mangetouts
    with Miso
Sautéed Red and Yellow Peppers
Steamed New Potatoes with
    Herbs
Tossed Mixed Green Salad
Apple Crisp

Saturday

Breakfast
Mixed-grains Porridge with Fruit
4fl. oz (120ml) orange juice or
    ½ grapefruit

Lunch
Warm Chick-pea Salad
Wholemeal bread
1 piece fruit, or Oranges with Figs

Dinner
Pasta with Uncooked Tomatoes
Tossed Mixed Green Salad
Peach Cobbler

Sunday

Breakfast
Wholemeal toast with Apricot or
    Apple Purée
4fl. oz (120ml) orange juice or
    ½ grapefruit

Lunch
Puréed Pumpkin Soup
Tossed Mixed Green Salad
Fruit Salad

Dinner
Grilled Tofu 'Cutlets'
Courgettes Provençale
Cooked grains of your choice
Watercress and Mushroom Salad
Apples with Lime Juice

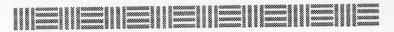

Monday

Breakfast
Unsweetened muesli with apple
   juice
4fl. oz (120ml) orange juice

Lunch
Indian Split-pea Soup
Wholemeal bread
1 piece fruit

Dinner
Stir-fried Tofu and Vegetables
Brown rice or millet
Oriental Beansprout Salad
Apple Purée

Tuesday

Breakfast
Mixed-grains Porridge
1 banana
4fl. oz (120ml) orange juice

Lunch
Miso Soup
Tossed Mixed Green Salad
Wholemeal bread

Dinner
Curried Brown Rice Salad
Aubergine Purée on wholemeal
   bread
Strawberry Ice
Wednesday

Breakfast
Mixed-grains Porridge with Fruit
4fl. oz (120ml) orange juice

Lunch
Pizza Sandwich (omit cheese; top
   with tofu, if desired)
Tossed Mixed Green Salad
1 piece fruit

Dinner
Potato–Leek Soup
Broccoli Salad
Baked Tomatoes, or Tomato
   Salad
Fresh Fruit

Thursday

Breakfast
Unsweetened muesli with apple
   juice
4fl. oz (120ml) orange juice or
   1/2 grapefruit

Lunch
Watercress and Mushroom Salad
   with tofu added, if desired
Wholemeal bread
1 piece fruit

Dinner
Black-bean Burritos (omit cheese)
Spinach Salad
Baked Apples

Friday

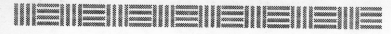

Friday

Breakfast
Wholemeal toast with Apple
  Purée
1 banana
4fl. oz (120ml) orange juice

Lunch
Chilled Tofu with Dipping Sauces
Wholemeal bread
1 piece fruit

Dinner
Hot and Sour Soup (omit egg)
Spicy Aubergines and Mangetouts
  with Miso
Cooked bulgur or millet
Pear Compôte

Saturday

Breakfast
Couscous with Fruit
4fl. oz (120ml) orange juice

Lunch
Tabouli
Tomato Salad

Dinner
Grated Carrot Salad
Vegetable Couscous
Oranges with Figs

Sunday

Breakfast
Wholemeal Bagels with Apple
  Purée
Fruit Salad

Lunch
Black-eyed Beans with Tomatoes
  and Herbs
Tossed Mixed Green Salad

Dinner
Beetroot and Vegetable Borscht
Marinated Vegetables
Orange Ice

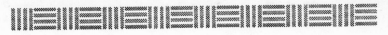

Week 3

Monday

Breakfast
Mixed-grains Porridge
4fl. oz (120ml) orange juice

Lunch
Marinated Vegetable pittas
1 piece fruit

Dinner
Indian Chick-pea Soup, or Warm
    Chick-pea Salad
Tossed Mixed Green Salad
Apple Crisp

Tuesday

Breakfast
Unsweetened muesli with apple
    juice
4fl. oz (120ml) orange juice

Lunch
Grated Carrot Salad
Wholemeal bread
1 piece fruit

Dinner
Pizza (omit cheese)
Grilled Mushrooms
Spinach Salad
Poached Bananas

Wednesday

Breakfast
2 slices wholemeal toast with
    Apple or Apricot Purée
4fl. oz (120ml) orange juice or
    ½ grapefruit

Lunch
Warm Potato Salad
Sliced tomatoes
1 piece fruit

Dinner
Curried Tofu and Vegetables
    (omit yoghurt)
Saffron Millet
Tossed Mixed Green Salad
Apple Purée

Thursday

Breakfast
Fruity Oatmeal
4fl. oz (120ml) orange juice

Lunch
Lentil Salad
Wholemeal bread

Dinner
Hearty Mushroom and Barley
    Soup
Wholemeal bread
Broccoli Salad
Baked Pears

Friday

Breakfast
2 pieces wholemeal bread with
   Apple Purée
1 banana
4fl. oz (120ml) orange juice

Lunch
Courgette Soup with Dill
Tossed Mixed Green Salad
Wholemeal bread
1 piece fruit

Dinner
Pasta with Broccoli and Tomato
   Sauce
Spinach and Tangerine Salad
Dried Fruit Compôte

Saturday

Breakfast
Wholemeal Bagels with Apricot
   Purée
4fl. oz (120ml) orange juice

Lunch
Warm Vegetable Salad Sandwich
   or Pitta Pocket
1 piece fruit

Dinner
Black-eyed Beans with Tomatoes
Kasha
Tossed Mixed Green Salad or
   Spinach Salad
Strawberry Ice

Sunday

Breakfast
Mixed-grains Porridge with Fruit
4fl. oz (120ml) orange juice

Lunch
Millet–Lentil Salad
Sliced tomatoes
Apple Purée

Dinner
Minestrone (omit cheese)
Tossed Mixed Green Salad
Wholemeal bread
Orange Ice

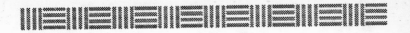

A Quick Weight-loss Plan

This diet plan doesn't differ too much from the preceding ones, except that I have cut out most of the lunchtime fruit or desserts and reduced the amount of bread. If you want even quicker results, reduce portions and cut the desserts from the dinner menus.

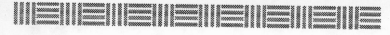

Week 1

Monday

Breakfast
Mixed-grains Porridge with Fruit
4fl. oz (120ml) orange juice

Lunch
Low-fat Egg Salad
Crudités

Dinner
Tofu with Dipping Sauces
Italian-style Spinach
Tossed Mixed Green Salad
Raspberry Ice

Tuesday

Breakfast
1 piece wholemeal bread spread
    with 1 tablespoon *fromage
    blanc* or low-fat cottage cheese
1 banana
4fl. oz (120ml) orange juice

Lunch
Carrot–Apple Salad
Sliced tomatoes

Dinner
Meatless Chilli
Spinach Salad
Orange with Mint

Wednesday

Breakfast
Unsweetened muesli with
    skimmed milk
4fl. oz (120ml) orange juice

Lunch
'Chillidog'
Tossed Mixed Green Salad

Dinner
Grilled Chicken Breasts
Watercress and Mushroom Salad
Sliced tomatoes
Apple Purée with natural low-fat
    yoghurt

Thursday

Breakfast
Scrambled Eggs
Wholemeal toast
4fl. oz (120ml) orange juice

Lunch
Blender Gazpacho
1 piece fruit

Dinner
Fish au Gros Sel
Middle Eastern Salad
Orange Ice

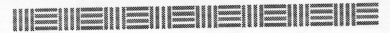

Friday

Breakfast
Fruity Oatmeal
4fl. oz (120ml) orange juice

Lunch
Tofu Salad
Crudités

Dinner
Piperade
Tossed Mixed Green Salad
Baked Apples

Saturday

Breakfast
Buckwheat Pancakes with Apple
    Purée and natural low-fat
    yoghurt (2 pancakes per
    serving)
4fl. oz (120ml) orange juice or
    ½ grapefruit

Lunch
Courgette Soup with Dill
1 piece fruit, or Oranges with
    Mint

Dinner
Stir-fried Tofu with Mangetouts
Bulgur (3oz/85g serving)
Tossed Mixed Green Salad
1 piece fruit

Sunday

Breakfast
Apple Omelette
4fl. oz (120ml) orange juice or
    ½ grapefruit

Lunch
Tabouli
Crudités

Dinner
Chicken Breasts Baked in Foil
Courgettes Provençale
Watercress and Mushroom Salad
Apples with Lime Juice

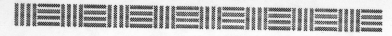

Week 2

Monday

Breakfast
Unsweetened muesli with
    skimmed milk and/or apple
    juice
4fl. oz (120ml) orange juice

Lunch
Chilled Cucumber Soup
1 piece fruit

Dinner
Stir-fried Tofu and Vegetables or
    Cod Fillets with Tomato–Mint
    Sauce
Brown rice or millet (3oz/85g
    portion)
Apple Purée

Tuesday

Breakfast
Banana Smoothie

Lunch
Cottage Cheese and Fruit Salad

Dinner
Curried Brown Rice Salad
Aubergine Purée on sliced
    cucumbers
Strawberry Ice

Wednesday

Breakfast
Mixed-grains Porridge with Fruit
4fl. oz (120ml) orange juice

Lunch
Sliced tomatoes
Lentil Salad

Dinner
Potato–Leek Soup
Tossed Mixed Green Salad
Frozen Apple Yoghurt

Thursday

Breakfast
1 soft-boiled egg
1 slice wholemeal toast
4fl. oz (120ml) orange juice or
    ½ grapefruit

Lunch
Low-fat cottage cheese
Watercress and Mushroom Salad

Dinner
Rabbit Cooked in Chicken Stock
    and Wine with Fresh Peas
Spinach Salad
Baked Apples

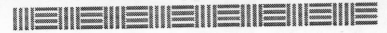

Friday

Breakfast
Unsweetened muesli with
    skimmed milk
4fl. oz (120ml) orange juice

Lunch
Spinach and Tofu Pitta
1 piece fruit

Dinner
Hot and Sour Soup
Oriental Beansprout Salad
Orange Ice

Saturday

Breakfast
Cottage Cheese–Apple Pancakes
    with Apple Purée
4fl. oz (120ml) orange juice

Lunch
Blender Gazpacho
1 piece fruit

Dinner
Grated Carrot Salad
Grilled Sole
Oranges with Mint

Sunday

Breakfast
Wholemeal Bagels with Low-fat
    Cream Cheese
Fruit Salad

Lunch
Apple Omelette
Tossed Mixed Green Salad

Dinner
Beetroot and Vegetable Borscht
Marinated Vegetables
1 piece fruit

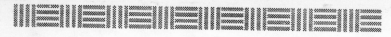

Week 3

Monday

Breakfast
6fl. oz (180ml) natural low-fat
   yoghurt with 1 tablespoon
   Apricot Purée
1 slice wholemeal toast spread
   with Apricot Purée
4fl. oz (120ml) orange juice

Lunch
Marinated Vegetable pittas

Dinner
Spicy Chick-pea Soup
Tossed Mixed Green Salad
Strawberry or Raspberry Ice

Tuesday

Breakfast
Unsweetened muesli with
   skimmed milk
4fl. oz (120ml) orange juice

Lunch
Low-fat Egg Salad or Salad Niçoise
1 piece fruit

Dinner
Pizza
Grilled Mushrooms
Spinach Salad

Wednesday

Breakfast
1 soft-boiled egg
1 slice wholemeal toast
4fl. oz (120ml) orange juice or
   ½ grapefruit

Lunch
Oriental Beansprout Salad
Sliced tomatoes
1 piece fruit

Dinner
Curried Tofu and Vegetables or
   Grilled Chicken Breasts with
   Tarragon
Saffron Millet (3oz/85g servings)
Tossed Mixed Green Salad
Apple Purée

Thursday

Breakfast
Fruity Oatmeal
4fl. oz (120ml) orange juice

Lunch
Cottage Cheese and Fruit Salad

Dinner
Hearty Mushroom and Barley
   Soup
Broccoli Salad
Baked Pears

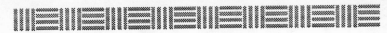

Friday

Breakfast
1 piece wholemeal bread spread
  with 1 tablespoon Low-fat
  Cream Cheese, *fromage blanc*
  or low-fat cottage cheese
1 banana
4fl. oz (120ml) orange juice

Lunch
Courgette Soup with Dill or
  Blender Gazpacho
Tossed Mixed Green Salad

Dinner
Grilled Salmon Steaks
Spinach and Tangerine Salad
Natural low-fat yoghurt with
  Apricot Purée

Saturday

Breakfast
Wholemeal Waffles with natural
  low-fat yoghurt and Apricot
  Purée
4fl. oz (120ml) orange juice

Lunch
Tofu Salad
Crudités
1 piece fruit

Dinner
Provençal Garlic Soup
Tossed Mixed Green Salad, or
  Spinach Salad
Baked Pears

Sunday

Breakfast
Scrambled Eggs
1 slice wholemeal toast with
  fromage blanc

Lunch
Broccoli Salad
Sliced tomatoes
Apple Purée

Dinner
Minestrone or Sweet and Sour
  Prawn
Tossed Mixed Green Salad
Wholemeal bread
Orange Ice

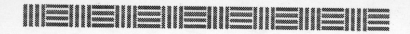

Quick Meals and Advice for Saving Time

It is true that a diet that involves chopping and cutting is more time-consuming than one that requires little more than throwing a chop in a pan. But several recipes in this book are really quite easy to prepare, and have quick cooking times. Grains and pulses take a while to cook, but this is passive cooking time: you are not required to be at the cooker, stirring and supervising. Also, many of these items can be prepared in advance and kept for several days in the refrigerator. When you are making a batch of rice, say, or beans or potatoes, double the quantity and use it in different dishes over the next few days. You can also use tinned beans for many of the recipes in the book, especially the salads.

Advance vegetable preparation

You can prepare many of your vegetables for soups, salads and vegetable dishes in advance and store them separately in sealed plastic bags or containers. They will keep for several days in the fridge if properly stored. Here are some suggestions.

onions: chop.

garlic: peel cloves and leave whole.

carrots: peel.

green peppers: chop some, cut others into strips.

parsley: wash, dry and chop.

lettuce: separate leaves, wash, dry and wrap in kitchen towels. Refrigerate in sealed plastic bags.

cucumbers: chop or slice, according to recipes.

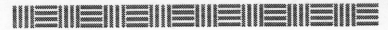

courgettes: slice.

broccoli and cauliflower: break into florets.

celery: slice.

spinach: wash, stem, dry, wrap in paper towels. Refrigerate in sealed plastic bags.

salad dressing: make enough low-fat vinaigrettes (see pp. 53–4) for the week.

vegetable stock: make enough stock for the week and freeze or refrigerate (see p. 80).

grains and pulses: you can cook grains and beans up to three days ahead of time and store them in the refrigerator in covered containers, so they will be ready when you need them. Grains and cooked beans also freeze well.

A selection of quick menus

Low-fat Egg Salad
Wholemeal bread
1 piece fruit

Lentil Salad made with leftover
    lentils
Sliced tomatoes
Fruit

'Chilidogs' made with leftover chilli
Tossed Mixed Green Salad
1 piece fruit

Provençal Garlic Soup
Wholemeal bread
Broccoli Salad
Apple Purée with natural low-fat
    yoghurt

Scrambled Eggs
Wholemeal toast
Fruit

Blender Gazpacho
Wholemeal bread
Fruit Salad

Piperade
Steamed New Potatoes with
    Herbs
Tossed Mixed Green Salad
Apples with Lime Juice

Warm Chick-pea Salad made
    with tinned or leftover chick peas
Wholemeal bread
1 piece fruit, or Oranges with Figs

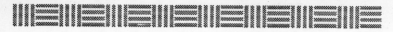

Pasta with Uncooked Tomatoes
Tossed Mixed Green Salad
Fruit

Grilled Tofu 'Cutlets'
Steamed green vegetable
Couscous or bulgur
Apples with Lime Juice

Chilled Cucumber Soup
Wholemeal bread
Fruit

Cottage Cheese and Fruit Salad
Wholemeal Bread

Curried Brown Rice Salad made
   with leftover rice
Wholemeal bread
Fruit

Pizza Sandwich made with left-
   over tomato sauce
Tossed Mixed Green Salad
Fruit

Potato–Leek Soup
Baked Tomatoes
Tossed Mixed Green Salad
Fruit

Low-fat cottage cheese
Watercress and Mushroom Salad
Wholemeal bread
Fruit

Spinach and Tofu Pitta Sandwich
Fruit

Hot and Sour Soup
Oriental Beansprout Salad
Fruit

Marinated Vegetable pittas made
   with leftover Marinated
   Vegetables
Fruit

Spaghetti with Simple Tomato
   Sauce
Grilled Mushrooms
Spinach Salad
Banana–Yoghurt Ice-cream

Hearty Mushroom and Barley
   Soup
Wholemeal bread
Tomato Salad
Baked Pears

Courgette Soup with Dill
Tossed Mixed Green Salad
Wholemeal bread
Fruit

Pasta with Broccoli and Tomato
   Sauce
Spinach and Tangerine Salad
Yoghurt with Berries or Apricot
   Purée

Chilled Tofu with Dipping Sauces
Spinach and Tangerine Salad
Baked Apples

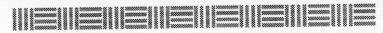

Mushroom Omelette
Wholemeal bread
Steamed green vegetable
Tossed Mixed Green Salad
Fruit

American Southern Spoonbread
Sautéed Okra with Tomatoes
Tossed Mixed Green Salad
Fruit

Mixed Bean Salad made with
    tinned beans
Wholemeal bread
Fruit

Cabbage Soup Chinoise
Carrot–Apple Salad (use food
    processor)
Wholemeal bread
Fruit

Miso Soup
Tossed Mixed Green Salad
Wholemeal bread
Fruit

Puréed Potato and Parsley Soup
Batavia and Orange Salad
Fruit

Any of the following as a main dish:

Grilled Chicken Breasts
Grilled Chicken Breasts with
    Tarragon
Chicken Breasts Baked in Foil
Fish Fillets Grilled in Foil with
    Garlic and Mushrooms
Grilled Sole
Cod with Tomato–Mint Sauce

accompanied by:

Steamed New Potatoes with
    Herbs or Couscous
Steamed green vegetable
Tossed Mixed Green Salad
Fresh fruit

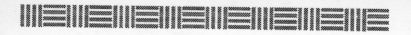

Low-sodium Diets

People suffering from hypertension need to reduce or eliminate their salt intake. The recipes in this book, so many of which are based on vegetables which have an inherent good flavour and require no salt anyway, adapt well to low-sodium diets. Almost all of them contain fresh herbs and/or spices, which add flavour and zest. Grains have a very nutty taste of their own. I find that vinegar and lemon juice enhance many saltless dishes. Salt is actually an acquired taste, and once you eliminate it from your diet you will quickly lose your desire for it and begin actually to taste the food.

There are, however, some foods that taste very bland indeed without salt. Broth-based soups, some bean dishes and tofu are the first that come to mind. But some soups – for example vegetable purées such as Gazpacho (p. 107) – can taste fine in their saltless versions. You may want to pep up Gazpacho with a little more basil or lemon juice or a touch of vinegar. Many beans are bland without salt, but I find that chick peas, black-eyed beans and lentils all have strong enough flavours on their own, especially when cooked with tomatoes, garlic, herbs and spices. Tofu, on the other hand, is difficult to handle without a little soy sauce, so you may prefer to focus on the other recipes in this book. There are plenty to choose from.

Below is a list of recipes that best adapt to a low-sodium diet. All you need to do is eliminate the salt and/or soy sauce.

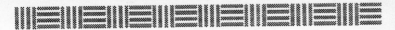

Suggested alternative seasonings

fresh herbs
cayenne
cumin
freshly ground black pepper
mustard

cider or wine vinegar
fresh lemon juice
lemon rind
orange peel

Breakfasts

Apple Omelette
Buckwheat Pancakes
Couscous with Fruit
Fruity Oatmeal
Low-fat Blender Drinks

Mixed-grains Porridge
Mixed-grains Porridge with Fruit
Oatmeal Pancakes
Scrambled Eggs
Wholemeal Waffles

Breads

Apple–Raisin Muffins
Banana–Nut Muffins
Blueberry Rice Muffins
Bran Muffins

Cranberry Muffins
Orange–Apricot Muffins
Sweet Potato Muffins

Spreads, dressings, sauces, purées, condiments

Apple Purée
Apricot Purée
Aubergine Purée
Haricot Bean Purée
Humous

Low-fat Salad Dressings (except
    Tofu Mayonnaise)
Prune Butter
Salsa Fresca

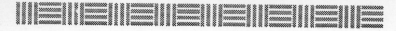

Sandwiches

'Chilidogs'
Marinated Vegetable Pittas

Pizza Sandwiches
Warm Vegetable Salad
    Sandwiches or Pitta Pockets

Salads

Batavia and Orange Salad
Broccoli Salad
Bulgur Pilaf Salad
Carrot–Apple Rice Salad
Curried Brown Rice Salad
Grated Carrot Salad
Lentil Salad
Marinated Vegetables
Mexican Corn Salad
Mexican Rice Salad
Middle Eastern Salad

Mixed Bean Salad
Oriental Beansprout Salad
Spinach Salad
Spinach and Tangerine Salad
Tabouli
Tomato Salad
Tossed Mixed Green Salad
Warm Chick-pea Salad
Warm Potato Salad
Warm Vegetable Salad
Watercress and Mushroom
    Salad

Soups

Bean and Vegetable Soup
Blender Gazpacho
Chick-pea Soup
Chilled Cucumber Soup
Corn Chowder
Curried Cabbage and Apple
    Soup

Fresh Pea Soup
Hearty Lentil Soup
Hearty Mushroom and Barley
    Soup
Indian Split-pea Soup
Minestrone
Split-pea Soup

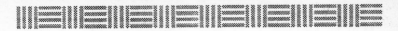

Fish and chicken dishes

Chicken and Vegetable Curry
Grilled Chicken Breasts
Steamed Fillets of Sole with
 Tomato Sauce
Grilled Sole
Cod Fillets with Tomato–Mint
 Sauce

Fish Fillets Grilled in Foil with
 Garlic and Mushrooms
Fillets of Sole with Cucumbers
 and Dill
Grilled Chicken Breasts with
 Tarragon

Vegetarian main dishes

Baked Potatoes with Low-fat
 Toppings
Black-eyed Beans with
 Tomatoes and Herbs
Curried Tofu and Vegetables
Meatless Chilli
Mushroom Omelette
Mushroom Toasts
Pasta with Aubergine and
 Tomato Sauce
Pasta with Broccoli and Tomato
 Sauce

Pasta with Creamy Tomato
 Sauce
Pasta with Uncooked Tomatoes
Piperade
Pizza
Soft Potato–Bean Tacos
Spicy Green Beans
Spinach Lasagne
Spaghetti with Simple Tomato
 Sauce
Vegetable Couscous

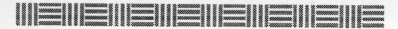

Grains and pulses

(Season further with a splash of vinegar or freshly squeezed lemon juice)

Bulgur Pilaf
Chick Peas with Spinach
Courgette and Rice Terrine
Greek-style Haricots
Italian Rice-stuffed Tomatoes
Kasha with Vegetables
Lentil and Bulgur Pilaf

Middle Eastern Lentils with
    Vegetables
North Indian Pilaf
Savoury Haricot Beans
    Provençale
Wild Rice and Mushroom Pilaf

Vegetable side-dishes

Baked Tomatoes
Baked Yams or Sweet Potatoes with
    Lime
Cucumbers Simmered in White
    Wine
Courgettes Provençale
Curried Pumpkin Purée
Fresh Peas with Mint and Lettuce
Grilled Mushrooms
Italian-style Spinach
Potato Gratin

Pumpkin and Sweet Potato
    Purée
Sautéed Okra and Tomatoes
Sautéed Red and Yellow Peppers
Spiced Vegetables en Papillote
Steamed Artichokes with Low-
    fat Yoghurt Dressing
Steamed Greens with Vinegar or
    Lemon Juice
Steamed New Potatoes with
    Herbs
Steamed Peas and Cauliflower

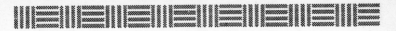

Desserts

Apple Crisp
Apple Purée
Apples with Lime Juice
Baked Apples
Baked Pears
Banana–Yoghurt Ice-cream
Brown Rice Pudding
Cheesecake
Dried Fruit Compôte
Frozen Apple Yoghurt
Frozen Yoghurt Lollies
Fruit Salads

Millet Raisin Pudding
Noodle Kugel
Oatmeal Raisin Biscuits
Orange Ice
Oranges with Figs
Peach Cobbler
Pear Compôte
Poached Bananas
Strawberry or Raspberry Ice
Winter Fruit Ambrosia
Yoghurt with Berries

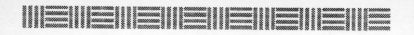

Suggestions for Pregnancy

Pregnancy is no time for dieting. During these nine months your protein requirements increase by 75 per cent, your calcium and iron requirements by about 50 per cent. You need to obtain lots of B vitamins, vitamin C and vitamin A. In short, you need to eat more.

This is when there is no room for empty calories. Every calorie has to count. The nice thing about the recipes in this book is that they are so low in fat that increasing your calorific intake in order to increase protein, vitamin and mineral consumption will not add an undue amount of fat to your diet. In fact, a small increase in fat may be necessary in order for you to get enough vitamin E. Olive oil and wheatgerm are good sources.

Because your appetite may not be very good during pregnancy, and as the months go by you may not be able to eat much at one time, you might want to eat several small meals throughout the day rather than three big ones. Mid-morning and mid-afternoon snacks provide you with good opportunities for obtaining the necessary nutrients.

The following foods provide valuable nutrients during pregnancy:

dairy products: protein, calcium, vitamin D.

eggs: protein, vitamin A, zinc.

grains, wholemeal breads and cereals: iron, B vitamins, minerals, protein (must be eaten in combination with beans or dairy products to obtain complete protein), fibre.

pulses: protein, fibre, iron, magnesium.

leafy green vegetables: B vitamins, magnesium.

dark leafy greens, broccoli: calcium, B vitamins, vitamin A.

carrots: vitamin A.

potatoes: minerals, B vitamins.

fish, rabbit, chicken and turkey without the skin: good protein with very little fat.

dried fruit: iron, potassium.

citrus fruit: vitamin C.

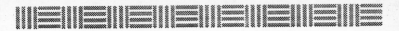

Five high-protein breakfasts

Mixed-grains Porridge with 8fl. oz
    (225ml) skimmed milk
8fl oz (225ml) orange juice

Scrambled Eggs
2 slices wholemeal toast with
    fromage blanc
½ grapefruit or 8fl. oz (225ml)
    orange juice

Cottage Cheese–Apple Pancakes
    with Low-fat Yoghurt Topping
Melon or orange juice

Unsweetened muesli with 8fl. oz
    (225ml) skimmed milk or
    natural low-fat yoghurt
Melon or orange juice

Apple Omelette
2 slices wholemeal toast with
    fromage blanc
Orange juice

Six high-protein lunches

Try to drink 8fl. oz (225ml) skimmed milk, or eat the equivalent amount
of low-fat yoghurt with each lunch.

Spinach and Tofu Pitta Sandwiches
Crudités
Yoghurt with Berries

Cottage Cheese and Fruit Salad
1 slice wholemeal bread with
    fromage blanc
Frozen Apple Yoghurt

Tuna Salad Pitta Pockets
Crudités
Low-fat yoghurt
Fresh fruit

Tofu Salad Sandwich
Tossed Mixed Green Salad
1 orange

Chinese Chicken Salad
1 slice wholemeal bread with
    fromage blanc
Steamed broccoli
Fresh fruit

Low-fat Egg Salad sandwich
Broccoli Salad, or crudités
Fresh fruit

Note: You may add an ounce or two of cheese to these meals.

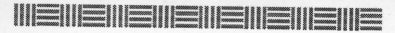

Ten high-protein vegetarian dinners

Broccoli Salad
Spicy Chick-pea Soup
Wholemeal bread
Dried Fruit Compôte with Low
    fat Yoghurt

Grated Carrot Salad
Spinach Lasagne
Wholemeal bread
Baked Tomatoes, or Grilled
    Mushrooms
Banana–Yoghurt Ice-cream

Oriental Beansprout Salad
Stir-fried Tofu with Mangetouts
Saffron Millet
Pumpkin Purée
Cheesecake

Piperade
Spiced Vegetables en Papillote
Wholemeal bread
Tossed Mixed Green Salad
Brown Rice Pudding

Spinach and Tangerine Salad
Hearty Lentil Soup
Wholemeal bread
Frozen Apple Yoghurt

Tofu Noodle Soup
Broccoli Timbale
Wholemeal bread
Baked Tomatoes
Tossed Mixed Green Salad
Strawberry Ice

Greek-style Haricots
Kasha with Vegetables
Steamed Greens with Vinegar or
    Lemon Juice
Wholemeal bread
Baked Apples with Low-fat
    Yoghurt

Curried Tofu and Vegetables
Brown rice
Carrot–Apple Salad
Yoghurt with Berries

Spinach Salad, or Broccoli Salad
Hearty Mushroom and Barley
    Soup
Wholemeal bread
Cheesecake

Courgette and Rice Terrine
Minestrone
Tossed Mixed Green Salad
Dried Fruit Compôte with Low-
    fat Yoghurt

Note: You may add an ounce or two of cheese to these meals.

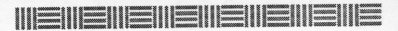

Ten high-protein dinners with fish, chicken and rabbit

Grilled Salmon Steaks
Steamed potatoes or whole grains
Baked Tomatoes
Spinach Salad
Fresh Fruit

Sweet and Sour Prawns
Brown rice
Steamed broccoli
Oriental Beansprouts Salad
Orange Ice

Grilled Sole
Steamed potatoes or whole grains
Italian-style Spinach
Tomato Salad
Fresh fruit

Grilled Chicken Breasts with
    Tarragon
Bulgur Pilaf
Steamed green beans
Grated Carrot Salad
Banana–Yoghurt Ice-cream

Rabbit Cooked in Chicken Stock
    and Wine with Fresh Peas
Fresh pasta
Tossed Mixed Green Salad
Oranges with Mint

Fillets of Sole with Cucumbers
    and Dill
Baked Tomatoes
Kasha
Tossed Mixed Green Salad
Fresh fruit

Chicken Breasts Baked in Foil
Steamed artichokes with Tofu
    Dressing
Tossed Mixed Green Salad
Strawberry Ice

Salade Niçoise
Wholemeal bread
1oz (30g) cheese
Banana–Yoghurt Ice-cream

Chicken and Vegetable Curry
Bulgur
Carrot–Apple Salad
Yoghurt with Berries

Steamed Cod Fillets with
    Tomato–Caper Sauce
Fresh pasta
Broccoli Salad
Fresh fruit

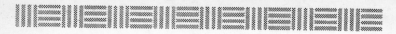

Between-meal snacks

Natural low-fat yoghurt with fruit or berries
Small portions of salads or leftovers from dinner
1–2 slices wholemeal bread with Cucumber–Cottage Cheese Spread
1–2 slices wholemeal bread with Haricot Bean Purée or Humous
Wholemeal Bagel with Low-fat Cream Cheese
Crudités with Low-fat Salad Dressing
Banana–Yoghurt Ice-cream
Millet Raisin Pudding
Brown Rice Pudding
Cheesecake
Any of the frozen yoghurt ice-lollies on pp. 215–17
Any of the blender drinks on pp. 42–5

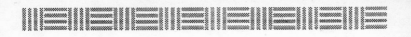

Menu Plans for Athletes

It is now widely accepted that athletes do not need to eat high-protein diets. In fact, they need to cut down on protein and emphasise complex carbohydrates. Muscles are fuelled by carbohydrates, which are stored in the muscles as a substance called *glycogen*. When muscles work they burn the glycogen; it must be resupplied several times during the day. That's just what a high-carbohydrate diet will do; it will double the amount of glycogen in your muscles and increase your energy supply.

These must be *complex* carbohydrates, like grains, cereals, potatoes and pasta – not confectionery and soft drinks. Complex carbohydrates are the key to regulating your metabolism and burning fats. Simple carbohydrates – sugar – stimulate the pancreas to produce high levels of insulin, which tells the body to make and store fat, and makes you get hungry more often. Sugar increases the level of fats in the blood, which reduces your athletic endurance and puts you at high risk for cardiovascular disease.

Protein does nothing to increase your energy supply, and in fact an unbalanced high-protein diet can reverse the effects of exercise and can be harmful for the athlete. The steak-and-eggs diet is not only a high-protein diet, it is a high-fat diet – much higher in calories than a high-carbohydrate diet. That's why we are finding more and more vegetarians among Olympic Gold Medallists and other professional athletes. At any rate, it isn't necessary to eat red meat to get high-quality protein. You find the same amino acids in poultry, fish, low-fat dairy products, eggs and balanced combinations of grains and legumes.

The importance of water

The best drink for the athlete is water. Inadequate hydration is the major cause of poor performance in sports. Sports nutritionists say that water is the athlete's single most important nutrient. The body needs it to regulate its temperature through perspiration, to rid itself of toxic wastes through urination and to maintain proper blood pressure. Water supplies the

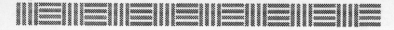

muscles and organs with oxygen and nutrients, and water is vital for the energy-supplying chemical reactions to occur in the muscles.

Thirst is not an adequate indication of how much water an active person needs. You need to force it. That's not too difficult if you begin to replace sugary sodas and 'sports drinks' with water. Athletes should drink at least ³/₄ pint (425ml) before exercise or competition, and should continually drink during competition. *Eat to Win* nutrition doctor Robert Haas recommends three or more glasses 3 hours prior to sports events, two glasses 60–15 minutes before, and at least two glasses per hour while performing. After the event he advises that you weigh yourself and drink two glasses of water for every pound you've lost. The more active you are, the more water you need.

The idea that athletes should take salt tablets is a myth that couldn't be further from the truth. Salt tablets are dangerous for anybody, and especially for athletes. They distort the ratio of salt and water in the body and interfere with the body's sweating mechanism. Too much salt can harm the kidneys. If you are worried about losing salt, drink more water.

What to eat

Active people, then, should forget what they've been told all their lives about potatoes, grains, pasta and (wholegrain) bread. These foods are not 'fattening', and they should constitute 65 per cent of your daily calorific intake. Grains and wholemeal breads are excellent sources of complex carbohydrates. They also supply lots of fibre and vitamins.

Other important nutrients for athletes are potassium, magnesium and thiamin. Potassium, abundant in bananas, dried fruits, nuts, orange juice and potatoes, helps regulate the water balance in the body and catalyses the release of energy and other muscle-cell activities. Insufficient potassium causes muscle fatigue and weakness. Magnesium, abundant in dark, leafy greens, whole grains, almonds and cashews, fish and milk, is necessary for proper muscle contraction and relaxation, as well as for energy release. Thiamin helps burn carbohydrates. Good sources of thiamin are whole grains and wholemeal breads, milk and eggs.

Women have greater iron needs than men, especially when involved in contact sports like basketball, martial arts and jogging (which jars like contact sports). This is because bruising causes hidden blood loss. Some

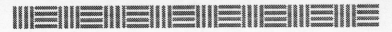

foods rich in iron are dried beans, fresh fruits, grains, broccoli and Brussels sprouts, and leafy green vegetables like spinach. Eating foods rich in vitamin C along with iron-rich foods will help you absorb the iron. Have an orange with your spinach salad. Calcium and riboflavin (vitamin B-2) are also important nutrients for active women. Dairy products, leafy green vegetables and broccoli, and dried beans are all high in calcium.

Men who are in training and need to gain weight should increase not their protein intake but their consumption of complex carbohydrates: more potatoes, more wholegrain bread. Wrestlers and participants in other weight-control sports often have severe nutritional problems because of fasting to 'make weight'. These athletes and their coaches need to review their attitudes about weight control, and their practices. Fasting depletes athletes of carbohydrate stores and water necessary for peak performance. If the athletes also take diuretics and cathartics they deplete their bodies of the minerals necessary for muscle function.

Maintenance diet for athletes

No matter what your sport is, the following menus will provide you with a diet low in fat and high in complex carbohydrates, vitamins and minerals. These menus are suitable for all active people, whether morning jogger or football-team captain. For those whose work-out needs require more calories, foods whose amounts can be increased are noted.

Five breakfasts

2–4 oz (55g–115g) unsweetened
  muesli
4fl. oz (120ml) skimmed milk
I banana
6fl. oz (180ml) orange juice

Scrambled Eggs
2 slices wholemeal toast
1/2 grapefruit
6fl. oz (180ml) orange juice

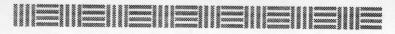

1 serving Fruity Oatmeal
4fl. oz (120ml) skimmed milk
4fl. oz (120ml) orange juice

2–3 Cottage Cheese–Apple
    Pancakes
Apple Purée
1 additional piece fruit
6fl. oz (180ml) orange juice

1 serving Noodle Kugel, or 2–3
    Buckwheat Pancakes with
    natural low-fat yoghurt and
    Apple Purée
1 additional piece fruit
6fl. oz (180ml) orange juice

If you feel you need more calories to sustain you: increase cereals by 1–2 oz
(30-55g); increase toast or pancakes by 1 serving.

Five lunches

Cucumber–Cottage Cheese
    Spread Sandwich on wholemeal
    bread
Crudités
Apple
8fl. oz (225ml) skimmed milk

Tofu Salad Sandwich
Crudités
Apple, pear or orange
Still or sparkling mineral water, or
    4fl. oz (120ml) skimmed milk

'Chilidog' with 1oz (30g) grated
    cheese
Crudités
Apple, pear or orange
Still or sparkling mineral water

Low-fat Egg Salad sandwich on
    wholemeal or pitta bread
Crudités
Apple, pear or orange
½oz (15g) cheese, or 4fl. oz
    (120ml) skimmed milk
Still or sparkling mineral water

Spinach and Tofu Pitta Sandwich
Crudités
Apple, pear or orange
Bran Muffin
4fl. oz (120ml) skimmed milk, or
    sparkling or still mineral water

If you feel you need more calories to sustain you: add more crudités to each
lunch, or 1 Bran Muffin, or 4fl. oz (120ml) natural low-fat yoghurt.

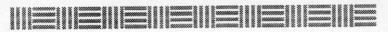

Five dinners

Hearty Lentil Soup
Spinach Salad
Wholemeal bread
Apple Crisp, or Frozen Apple
  Yoghurt

Mushroom Risotto
Wholemeal bread
Baked Tomatoes
Broccoli Salad
Dried Fruit Compôte

Meatless Chilli
Cornbread
Tossed Mixed Green Salad with
  Low-fat Vinaigrette
Steamed broccoli or courgettes
Noodle Kugel

Spaghetti with Simple Tomato
  Sauce and Parmesan
Wholemeal bread
Steamed green vegetable, or
  Italian-style Spinach
Tossed Mixed Green Salad with
  Low-fat Vinaigrette
Banana–Yoghurt Ice-cream

Grilled Tofu 'Cutlets'
Brown rice or Baked Potato with
  Low-fat Yoghurt Topping
Steamed broccoli, greens,
  courgettes or cauliflower
Tossed Mixed Green Salad with
  Low-fat Dressing
Baked Apples

If you feel you need more calories to sustain you: add crudités, as much as you desire, to each meal, or 1 slice wholemeal bread.

Pre-competition meals

The pre-competition meal should be small and simple, and should be eaten two hours before competition. Its goals are to provide your muscles with the energy they will need, to prevent hunger during competition, to hydrate the body and prevent gastro-intestinal upset. Eat meals high in complex carbohydrates and avoid fats. Drink lots of water – about 8fl. oz (225ml) for each 50 pounds of your body weight, and 8fl. oz (225ml) for each 15 minutes of strenuous physical activity that you will be engaging in.

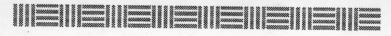

Competition-day diet

Five breakfasts

2 muffins (your choice, pp. 26–33)

4fl. oz (120ml) natural low-fat yoghurt, cottage cheese or skimmed milk

1 banana

2–3 large glasses water

2 slices wholemeal toast or wholemeal bagel

2 tablespoons Apple Purée

4fl. oz (120ml) natural low-fat yoghurt or cottage cheese

1 piece fruit

2–3 large glasses water

2oz (55g) unsweetened muesli with skimmed milk and/or apple juice

1 piece fruit

2–3 large glasses water

Banana–Yoghurt Smoothie, or 1 serving Brown Rice Pudding

1–2 Bran Muffins or slices wholemeal toast

1 portion Mixed-grains Porridge with Fruit

4fl. oz (120ml) skimmed milk

2–3 large glasses water

Five lunches

Marinated Vegetable pitta
Apple
2 oatmeal biscuits

Pasta with Creamy Tomato Sauce
Apple, banana or orange

Baked Potato with Low-fat Toppings
Apple, banana or orange

Tofu Salad Sandwich
2 Oatmeal Biscuits
Apple, banana or orange

8fl. oz natural low-fat yoghurt, or 6oz (140g) low-fat cottage cheese
Crudités
1 slice wholemeal bread
1 piece fruit

Liquid meals

(Good before evening competitions.)

Any of the blender drinks on pp. 42–5, accompanied by 1–2 muffins from pp. 26–33.

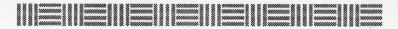

Post-competition meals

The purpose of the post-competition meal is to restore the glycogen burned by the muscles during exercise, and to replace the fluids, vitamins, minerals and protein the body has used up.

Five post-competition meals

These are very simple menus. You can, of course, depart from these and use the recipes in this book to make up more elaborate menus. The important thing here is to note the food items in each meal.

1 serving beans, 2 slices whole-
    meal bread or Cornbread
3oz (85g) steamed or raw green,
    yellow or orange vegetables
Tossed Mixed Green Salad or
    Spinach Salad (optional)
1 piece fruit
¾ pint (425ml) water, more as
    desired

1 serving beans, 1 serving cooked
    grains
1 slice wholemeal bread
3oz (85g) steamed or raw green,
    yellow or orange vegetables
Tossed Mixed Green Salad, or
    Spinach Salad (optional)
1 piece fruit
¾ pint (425ml) water, more as
    desired

1 serving cooked pasta or grains
    with tomato sauce
3oz (85g) steamed or raw green,
    yellow or orange vegetables
Tofu and Beansprout Salad
1 piece fruit
¾ pint (425ml) water, more as
    desired

1 serving beans, 6oz (170g) low-fat
    cottage cheese
3oz (85g) steamed or raw green,
    yellow or orange vegetables
Tossed Mixed Green Salad, or
    Spinach Salad (optional)
1 piece fruit
¾ pint (425ml) water, more as
    desired

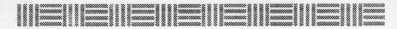

4oz (115g) serving Chilled Tofu
  with Dipping Sauces or soy
  sauce, or 2 eggs
1 Baked Potato with Low-fat
  Topping, or 2oz (55g) Wholemeal Pasta with Simple Tomato
  Sauce
3oz (85g) steamed or raw green,
  yellow or orange vegetables
1 piece fruit
³/₄ pint (425ml) water, more as
  desired

Note   For high-protein meals, substitute chicken, fish or rabbit for beans.

Eating in restaurants

Travelling to sports events necessitates eating in restaurants. But you can
still stick to a high-carbohydrate, low-fat diet. At almost all restaurants you
can find pasta, rice, baked potatoes, fish without butter, vegetables, salads
and fruit. Ask for potatoes, vegetables and grains without butter. Eat salads, but ask for the dressing on the side, and use the minimum. Or, even
better, ask the waiter for a lemon and season your salad with freshly
squeezed lemon juice (better tasting by far than the often rancid bottled
salad dressings chain restaurants usually offer). Salad bars are becoming
more and more common, and here is where you can really go to town.
Pile your plate with vegetables, chick peas, bean salads and cottage
cheese. But stay away from the creamy dressings. At pizza places you can
always order small pizzas and remove most of the cheese.

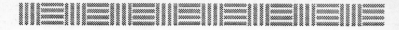

Acceptable restaurant meals

Baked potato with low-fat
  yoghurt, cottage cheese or
  mustard
Mixed green salad with lemon
  juice
Fresh fruit

Spaghetti with tomato sauce
Mixed green salad with lemon
  juice
Fresh fruit

Cottage cheese and fruit salad
Wholemeal bread (1–2 slices)
Black-bean burritos with lettuce
  and tomato
Mixed green salad, or spinach
  salad with lemon juice
Fresh fruit

Salad bar: vegetables, beans,
  cottage cheese, beansprouts,
  chopped egg, tuna, etc., but toss
  with vinegar or lemon juice
Wholemeal bread (1–2 slices)
Fresh fruit

Spinach salad with chopped eggs
  (ask for it without bacon),
  tossed with lemon juice
Wholemeal bread (1–2 slices)
Fresh fruit

Small pizza with no extra cheese
  or sausage, but with any
  combination of vegetables
Mixed green salad with lemon
  juice
Fresh fruit

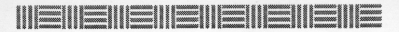

Index

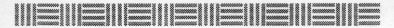

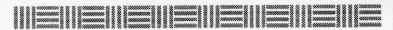

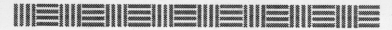

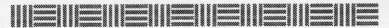

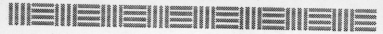